The
BIG
Vitamin
Dictionary

Michael LeVesque

Second Edition
Revised and Expanded
September 1, 2002

Lorren Daro Productions
Cobb Mountain, California

www.BIGvitamindictionary.com

= =   = =

The BIG Vitamin Dictionary
Copyright © 2002 by
Michael LeVesque
All Rights Reserved

ISBN: 0-9706608-2-0

Disclaimer: The contents of this book are based on the research of the author and are presented for educational purposes only. It is not a claim for a cure or mitigation of a disease, and it is not intended as medical advice. It is not intended to diagnose, treat, or prescribe for an illness. The author and the publisher are not responsible for any adverse effects or consequences resulting from the use of any of the products or preparations presented in this book. Health information cannot replace a health-care practitioner/patient relationship. Consumers should always consult with a health-care professional/practitioner for diagnosis and treatment of their specific health problems. This book is a discussion of nutrients found in the marketplace. To gain a deeper perspective regarding any of the entries, it is suggested that one consult some of the many other books published on these subjects.

Lorren Daro Productions
P.O. Box 9
Cobb, CA 95426

On the Internet:
www.BIGvitamindictionary.com

Table of Contents

Dedication

This book is dedicated in memory of Adele Davis, Paavo Airola, Carleton Fredericks, and Brian Leibowitz, who were great advocates of health, and shared their knowledge of nutrition.

Second, to the authors who have held a major place in providing nutritional information for the public, especially, Earl Mindell, Linda Rector-Page, James and Phyllis Balch, Michael Murray, Janet Zand, Paul Barney, Rick Scalzo, Sandra Hills, and Joseph Marion.

Third, to the many authors of who have presented innovative perspectives on health. Some of these are Ray Peat, H. Rudolph Alsleben, Michael Rosenbaum, Jon Kaiser, Richard Kunin, Jonathan Rothchild, Natasha Trenev, Richard Passwater, Steven Levine, Clara Felix, Jeffrey Reinhardt, and Paul Schulik.

Fourth, to my editor, publisher, friend, and the only real reason this book came into existence, Lorren Daro.

Fifth, to all of my family, managers, employees, customers, and friends. Special thanks to Dan Milosevich for his inspired writing and Webmaster tasks. Special thanks, and a very special place in my heart, to my proofreader, Camilla Lee.

Finally, special thanks to my daughters, Sarah, and especially Anna, the family nutritionist, for her in-depth editing and suggestions.

Have great health and a long life!

Michael LeVesque
San Francisco, California
June, 2002

PREFACE

Let the buyer be informed!

Throughout this book you will find statements about the curative abilities of nutritional supplements. **These statements are not to be taken as prescribing a cure!** There is a great difference. The preventative ability of these dietary supplements may stop the acquisition of a diseased state, however, once a person has had a definable disease diagnosed, the next step requires the intervention of a health-care practitioner. Whether dietary supplements will remain a high priority will be determined by the health-care practitioner's orientation. So choose wisely, for the use of pharmaceutical drugs can be an alternative that requires much higher levels of nutrients than will be presented in this small book. Also, try to find a practitioner who has an appreciation and knowledge of the nutritional benefits of dietary supplements, and their interactions with other drugs.

INTRODUCTION

Why take a supplement?

Some people, as they age, lose their health quickly, while others seem to never grow old. We can easily witness the effects of abuse due to alcohol and drugs, but it is much harder to recognize the ill-effects from sugar, bad fats and oils, and the lack of good nutrition. Of course, food, exercise, stress, culture, and genetics have their way with our health, but all of these cannot deny one very specific and important reality -- **life depends on nutrition!**

A healthy life depends on proper nutrition. In light of today's conditions, it is necessary to take nutritional supplements.

The body seeks health. Our performance and function depend on our chemical composition and what we supply to our body as nutrients. What we eat and drink are those nutrients. We also create nutrients within us. What we create depends on what we eat and drink.

Ideally, we want to eat and drink healthy things, reduce ineffective foods and drinks, and eliminate the harmful ones, but we don't have the knowledge or ability to analyze most of what we eat. We eat what is set before us. We have no control over the nutritional content of these items. Much worse is that we often eat things that appear good for us, but which are heavily laden with sugar, bad fats, extra salt, chemicals, and taste enhancers, which are, at best, void in nutrients, and at worst, dangerous. Also, we may not know that in most of the areas in which our foods are grown today, the soil may be very deficient in essential nutrients.

There is a continual barrage of chemicals in today's farming. Insecticides, disinfectants, fungicides, pesticides, herbicides, bactericides, virucides, antibiotics and hormones put us all at risk. We know that the residues of these chemicals create toxins and hormone imbalances. We also know that food changes from the time it is picked until the time we eat it. Food processing can result in a tremendous loss of essential nutrients.

Not one dietary survey has shown that Americans consume anywhere near the government RDA (Recommended Daily Allowance) of nutrients in their normal daily diets, even though these allowances are extremely small. Surveys consistently show that ignoring nutritional supplementation puts much of the American population at risk. Even the Journal of the American Medical Association recommends that everyone use nutritional supplements.

Americans of the 1900's ate food with much higher nutritive value than we do today. We are overfed and undernourished, and it is a national health problem. It is true that "food is our best medicine", and "we are what we eat", but if that food contains too many bad fats and empty calories, we find a great increase in the risk of heart disease. If the diet is too low in fiber and other important nutrients, we find a much higher risk of cancer. Obesity, our number one public health problem, creates a severe risk factor for high blood pressure, arthritis, heart disease, diabetes and cancer.

The overall nutrition we have available in the foods and beverages we eat and drink is inadequate. When something is inadequate you make up for it. You use the best information available and make a sensible choice -- you supplement the diet. Everyone in America today would greatly benefit from just taking a multiple vitamin and mineral tablet -- and, there are other important supplements, which you'll discover as we move along.

What is a vitamin?

Often we think of 'vitamin' as a general term for all the nutrients that we take to supplement our diet. But 'vitamin' only refers to very specific chemical compounds, such as riboflavin (B2) or niacin (B3) for example.

A vitamin is an essential organic catalytic substance. It acts as an ignition spark, which furnishes no fuel in itself, but keeps our fuel-burning system functioning in an orderly fashion. The fuel in question is the food we eat. To be labeled a vitamin, a substance must be shown to be essential to life and growth, and found to be necessary for maintaining proper bodily and reproductive health.

A substance can also be a crossover into other categories. For example, L-Carnitine is an amino acid compound, but because it fulfills the special definition of a vitamin, it is also called vitamin Bt. Another example is B3, or niacin, which has long been labeled a vitamin, but now it has the label of 'drug' because of its cholesterol-lowering activity.

Vitamin basics:

Fat-soluble vitamins are A, D, E, and K. They are stored in the fatty tissues, and have the potential for toxicity. The intestines, along with fats and lipids (oils) in foods, absorb them, and require protein to carry them along in the blood. They are not readily excreted, and are destroyed by free radicals.

Water-soluble vitamins include C, and all the separate B vitamins. These include choline, inositol, PABA (para-aminobenzoic acid), biotin, folic acid, pantothenic acid (B5), pyrodoxine (B6), thiamin (B1), and niacin (B3). These vitamins travel unattached in the lymph and blood systems, are easily flushed out in the urine, and are unlikely to cause toxicity.

Natural and synthetic vitamins have the same chemicals, but can differ in color and molecular structure. Natural vitamins tend to be more effective in most cases. This book will recommend the optimal form, synthetic or natural, when it will make a significant difference to your health and pocketbook.

What is a mineral?

Minerals and trace minerals (micro amounts of minerals), are the most basic of nutrients. They help you sleep, help your heart to beat, and keep your mind sharp and balanced. They are imperative for building and maintaining the integrity of your bones and tissues. They allow you to absorb other nutrients in the food you eat and transport them to your cells. They can only be obtained through foods and liquids, and cannot be synthesized by body chemistry. Minerals are inorganic substances which account for only four percent (4%) of body weight, yet they are the building blocks of life. The major minerals of the body are calcium, phosphorus, magnesium, potassium, sodium and chlorine.

The need for minerals is essential for life. Minerals work in combination with enzymes, hormones, and vitamins. They are essential for bone formation and energy production, especially for active people and athletes. Minerals participate in nerve transmission, muscle contraction and blood formation. More broadly, they regulate electrical activity in the nervous system, most of the metabolic functions of the body, and the osmosis of cellular fluids. People can tolerate a vitamin deficiency much longer than they can tolerate a deficiency in minerals.

Minerals cleanse the body, and can actually cure many diseases. The metabolic waste in the body is in the form of an acid. Minerals keep your body's pH in proper balance, so that it is alkaline instead of acid. The body unites the alkaline mineral with the waste acids and eliminates them through the urine. Some minerals compete with each other for absorption, while some enhance the absorption of other minerals. Some minerals work together, others do not.

How Minerals Interact with Each Other:

It is important to supplement with multiple mineral formulas rather than taking single minerals by themselves. However, after consulting with a health-care professional, certain medical conditions may require the supplementation of single minerals.

❑ Calcium depresses the absorption of magnesium, manganese, zinc and phosphorus.

- Phosphorus depresses the absorption of calcium, magnesium and iron.
- Magnesium depresses the absorption of phosphorus and calcium under certain circumstances, but enhances zinc and manganese.
- Sodium depresses the absorption of potassium, iron, copper, and cadmium, but enhances calcium, magnesium and manganese.
- Potassium depresses the absorption of sodium.
- Cadmium depresses the absorption of zinc and copper.
- Iron depresses the absorption of zinc, but enhances copper, molybdenum and cobalt.
- Zinc depresses the absorption of copper, magnesium, manganese, and cobalt, but enhances phosphorus and Vitamin B-1.
- Manganese depresses the absorption of calcium, phosphorus, iron and copper, but enhances, under certain circumstances, iron and copper.
- Copper depresses the absorption of zinc and manganese, but enhances iron, cobalt and Vitamin C.
- Molybdenum depresses the absorption of lead and Vitamin B-12.
- Selenium enhances the absorption of Vitamin E.

- Silicon enhances the absorption of calcium.
- Chlorine depresses the absorption of iron.
- Cobalt depresses the absorption of copper and enhances zinc, manganese, folic acid and Vitamin B-12.

How much Calcium to Magnesium?

It is not advisable to take a calcium or magnesium supplement by itself unless you are advised to do so by a health-care professional who is aware of certain mineral imbalances. In today's nutritional environment, it is suggested that the proper ratio of calcium to magnesium should be one-to-one. Premenstrual women require a ratio of two parts magnesium to one part calcium.

Recent research indicates that a magnesium deficiency causes reduced absorption of calcium, causing reduced calcium levels in the blood. Magnesium has a calcium-sparing effect, and decreases the need for calcium. Calcium also decreases the absorption of zinc; to offset this effect, it is important to supplement it, as well.

What about heavy metals?

Today, we are exposed to heavy metals such as cadmium, chlorine, aluminum, mercury, lead, and to toxic chemicals such as hydrocarbons and phenols. These environmentally-present toxins are a constant threat to health, and are almost impossible to avoid.

The use of certain nutrients can aid in the elimination of these toxins: Sulfur-containing amino acids such as cystine and methionine, sodium alginate, fruit pectin, manganese, zinc, iron, magnesium, iodine, Vitamin C, chlorophyll, MSM, and alpha lipoic acid.

Trace Minerals:

Trace minerals are one-tenth of one percent of body weight, yet deficiencies in these micronutrients can cause cancer, osteoporosis, depression, memory loss, high blood pressure, PMS, sugar imbalances (hypoglycemia and diabetes), premature aging, slow healing, and nerve disorders, to name but a few. The trace minerals include arsenic, chromium, cobalt, copper, fluoride, iodine, iron, manganese, molybdenum, nickel, selenium, silicon, tin, vanadium and zinc. The trace mineral list keeps growing as science discovers more about these micronutrients.

Why take a mineral supplement?

We don't get enough minerals. The most absorbable minerals are from fruits, vegetables and herbs. The pesticide sprays and chemical fertilizers used in commercial farming have created imbalances and have leached minerals from the soil.

This lack of good balanced minerals is also reduced by today's diet of processed foods, caffeine, and fatty foods. When we add high stress, the use of alcohol, tobacco, antibiotics, steroids, and industrial drugs, we find even more mineral depletion. We have only one alternative -- we must supplement them.

What is an amino acid?

Amino acids are the building blocks of protein. Presently, we have knowledge of about twenty-two amino acids of which our body is composed; of twenty others we know very little.

Amino acids are linked together by what are called peptide bonds to form over 1600 basic proteins. Each protein is composed of certain amino acids in a specific chemical

17

arrangement. Protein accounts for the majority of the solid weight of the body in the form of muscles, tendons, ligaments, organs, vital body fluids, glands, hair and nails.

Amino acids are an essential part of the body's growth, healing, and maintenance of health. The body uses amino acids in its hormone and enzyme systems, the lymph and blood, and in the formation of antibodies. Amino acids are necessary in the central nervous system as neurotransmitters, and are capable of crossing the blood brain barrier. They are necessary for keeping the proper pH levels in the body, providing energy to function, and in the formation of chromosomes. Also, amino acids are essential for the effectiveness of vitamins and minerals.

When we consume food that contains protein, the body digests it and breaks it down into amino acids. There are 'essential' amino acids, which the body cannot produce, and which it must get through the diet, and there are 'non-essential' amino acids produced by the liver through metabolic pathways that are also dependent on a sufficient supply of essential amino acids for their production. The body selects amino acids for building the proteins it requires. Therefore, amino acids, and not proteins, are considered the essential nutrients.

The liver produces about eighty percent of our amino acids, and the remainder must come from our diet. The quality of our diet is very important. Many elements can result in a deficiency of amino acids. The most common are poor diet, an imbalance of other nutrients, stress, trauma, drug use, poor digestion, infection, environmental pollution, and aging. A deficiency in amino acids can result in a multitude of problems, a few of which are anemia, depression, poor digestion, stunted growth, auto-immune disorders, neurological problems, muscle wasting, and ulcers. It is well-documented that many unspecific ailments and disease conditions are the result of the absence of certain amino acids in the body.

Amino acids come in three forms, but only the 'L' form is usually found on the shelves of the vitamin store. This is considered to be the 'natural' form, which is most easily absorbed by the body. Remember to take them, if possible, without food (especially proteins), and with extra water. Do not give them to children except under the guidance of a health-care provider.

What is an herb?

An herb is a plant food in which the bark, root, leaves, stems or flowers are used for health purposes. We possess knowledge of herbs from thousands of years of use, and billions of personal experiences. It is that great abundance of use and experience that led Hippocrates, the physician, to state, "Let your food be your medicine and your medicine be your food." The complex chemical compounds found in plants have far-reaching effects in the natural and safe healing of the body, yet they remain elusive to science.

Nevertheless, it was from plants that pharmaceutical drugs such as digitalis, aspirin and morphine were first derived. The goal was to reduce the herb to its most active ingredient, patent it, and get quick dependable results. Unfortunately, the reduction and isolation of certain chemical compounds has resulted in medicines that can have adverse effects on those who take them. We call these results 'side effects.' In reality, they are 'bad effects.'

The safety of whole herbs is well-documented, yet there is a legal struggle over declaring herbs a food or a drug. Certainly they are used in traditional medicine, and are the predominant form of medical treatment in the world today. The main criteria of herbs, however, should be their safety and purity from pesticides and chemicals, and not their medical efficacy. Herbs are agents of traditional medicine used to bring the body into balance and maintain health. They are not drugs. They are whole entities far too complex to reproduce in a laboratory. Herbs are a gift from nature, which appear to be most effective when used in their whole state, and not altered for an isolated active ingredient.

The use of herbs requires that you pay attention to your experience with them, and, when necessary, enlist the diagnosis of a qualified holistic physician or herbalist. The herbs listed in this book are only the popular ones that are most commonly found in stores. The information here is extremely abbreviated and requires further information if a person is taking a prescription drug, since some herbs interact with drugs.

There are many more herbs to get to know, so it's always good to have a reference book available for consultation. My suggestion is to begin with the earliest popular book on herbs in America, which is "Back to Eden" by Jethro Kloss, and can be found in most book stores across the country.

What are free-radicals?

Free-radicals are molecules with an unpaired electron that can damage cells. They are unstable and reactive, seeking to steal an electron from a nearby stable molecule that has paired electrons. Although free-radicals are necessary for life, an overabundance of free-radicals has been linked to heart disease, cancer, and other chronic degenerative diseases.

The body produces free-radicals through the metabolism of oxygen with various substances for energy, especially during times of illness and extreme stress, and through physical exercise. The environment produces free-radicals by way of air pollution, toxic waste, pesticides, herbicides, the sun's radiation, smoke, vehicle exhaust, food additives and certain medications.

Free-radicals can cause a chain reaction with other atoms resulting in cellular destruction. These free-radicals can damage the membrane tissue that holds cells together. This results in cell deterioration and the possible death of the cell. Free-radicals can damage protein structures such as RNA and DNA, the genetic material of the body, and consequently, cause your cells to produce deformed copies of themselves, making you age prematurely. They can break down molecules needed to keep your joints lubricated. Free-radicals can damage collagen, the substance that helps to hold the body together. They can narrow and close small arteries and capillaries, and can cause fats in the body to turn rancid and release more free-radicals.

What are antioxidants?

Antioxidants are a group of nutrients that are in our blood, organs, and all of our cells. They donate an electron to the free-radical and thereby neutralize it. These nutrients are not made in the body, but must be constantly supplied. Taken in sufficient amounts, antioxidants provide protection against free-radicals and the damage they can produce.

The major antioxidants are Vitamin A (beta-carotene), Vitamin C, Vitamin E, and selenium. There are many other nutrients that are antioxidants. These nutrients work best together and enhance each other's performance. Antioxidants can saturate our cells and provide protection at the cellular level against free radicals.

What is the immune system?

The immune system is our defense against foreign invaders such as bacteria, viruses, parasites, and other pathogens and toxins that cause the destruction of living cells. Infections are the results of these invaders, which can range from simple colds to debilitating illnesses such as cancer. Most diseases can be avoided by having a strong immune system.

The immune system is our body's only natural defense. It is composed of white blood cells, macrophages, antibodies, lymphatic tissue and the thymus gland. The immune system has the ability to adapt, learn, and remember its encounters with foreign invaders known as antigens. It carries a record of every antigen a person is exposed to, whether through breathing, eating, or contact with, or through, the skin.

The absence of even one component of the immune system can result in disease. This can occur due to heredity, birth defects, through illness, or produced by environmental factors, toxic chemicals, certain drug treatments, radiation, or from lack of proper nutrition.

Immunodeficiency disorders are a result of the immune system functioning inadequately, therefore, infections become more frequent, more severe, and last longer. They are a result of stress and malnutrition. Malnutrition may involve a deficiency of all nutrients, of primarily proteins, or of certain vitamins and minerals. Poor eating habits, coupled with food lacking in necessary nutrients, are a direct cause of immunodeficiency. Stress, resulting from day to day problems or traumatic events, affects both the body and the mind. This can cause depression, which can lower the immune response. Stress requires added nutrition.

The combination of toxic chemicals, environmental factors, certain drug therapies, and a state of malnutrition demand full attention to good nutrition as the key to defending the human body. Good nutrition eliminates and neutralizes many toxic environmental factors. Good nutrition eliminates the need for most drug therapies. Good nutrition neutralizes the affects of radiation. Good nutrition reduces the effects of stress on the body, and aids the mind's ability to cope with stress. Good nutrition reverses malnutrition.

Why <u>really</u> take supplements?

You take a supplement because you will benefit from it. You have to be patient. You have to be observant --

expectant, but not fooled. You have to maintain your objectivity in a subjective world. Practice paying attention to how you feel when you take supplements. Scientists have taken time to perform studies, run tests, and make judgements about these substances. It is now your turn to make your own judgements. You need to decide if you wish to continue using each of these supplements in your daily life. The longer you take a supplement, the more you will know if you like what it does for you. You may need to vary the dosage. You may need to take it over a period of time. Or, you may only have to take it once or twice to determine if you like the effects it produces.

What we ingest is directly correlated with a multitude of factors. It affects how we think, act, and perceive the world. Optimal nutrition has a definite place for everyone at every stage of his or her life. Ideally, awareness of one's personal nutritional needs should begin as early in life as possible. It is from this perspective that youthful arrogance develops into mature responsibility for one's health. Being knowledgeable about what your body needs to operate at the peak of energy, and in a state of health, is your means of maintaining optimum health far into a vital and vigorous old age.

How does it all work together?

Many nutrients can be synthesized in the body. Others, which are not synthesized in the body, must be supplied in the diet. Three elements are the trinity of optimum health: First, the essential amino acids must be supplied, along with fatty acids, vitamins and minerals. Second, antioxidants with their special function as free-radical scavengers are needed. Third, immune-system boosters to protect our bodies from disease.

Other components necessary for optimum health are fiber and friendly bacteria. There is also a vast array of miscellaneous compounds that are remedies for specific needs, disease conditions, and general enhanced performance. This category consists of herbs, elixirs, hormones, homeopathic remedies, enzymes, and certain chemicals. The entire nutritional system is very synergistic in that many of these substances, when taken together, increase each other's effectiveness.

Everything presented here is highly enhanced by your conscious state of awareness. Most of the time this is called the 'placebo' effect. However, what it also indicates is the mind's effect on the body, and its ability to initiate biochemical changes from a person's desires.

This powerful mental response is increased when the nutrients necessary to aid that change which the mind is conceiving are present in sufficient amounts to carry out that expectation.

Your intentions and attitude have a deep and lasting effect upon your health. The miracle of standing up and walking over to turn on a light switch is no greater or lesser than the miracle of curing a cancer within the human body. Maintaining optimum health is the goal. Good nutrition is the major key.

THE FIRST STEP TO NUTRITIONALLY OPTIMAL HEALTH

The very first step is to select a good, balanced, and complete multiple vitamin. For purposes of this discussion, I have created one formula, from many possible multiple vitamin and mineral formulas, to use as a model:

A Balanced Multi-Vitamin Formula:

Vitamin A 5,000IU
Beta Carotene 25,000IU/15mg
Vitamin B1 (thiamine) 100mg
Vitamin B2 (riboflavin) 100mg
Vitamin B3 (niacin) 100mg
Vitamin B6 (pyridoxine) 100mg
Vitamin B12 (cobalamin) 100mcg
Biotin 600mcg
Pantothenic Acid (Vitamin B5) 250mg
Choline 250mg
Inositol 250mg
PABA (para aminobenzoic acid) 50mg
Folic Acid (folate) 800mcg
Vitamin C (ascorbic acid) 1000mg
Vitamin D 400IU
Vitamin E 400IU
Calcium 1000mg
Magnesium 800mg
Potassium 100mg
Chromium 200mcg
Selenium 100mcg
Zinc 50mg

Manganese 5mg
Iron 20mg (for women)
Iron 30mg (for pregnant women)
Iron 10mg (for men)
Copper 2mg
Iodine 200mcg

Here are some additional nutrients one can add to approach <u>Super Nutrition</u>:

CoQ-10 100mg
Alpha Lipoic Acid 100mg
L-Carnitine 500mg
  or **Acetyl l-Carnitine** 500mg
L-Lysine 500mg
L-Proline 500mg
Omega-3 Oils 700mg
MSM 500mg
Pantethine 300mg
Bioflavonoids 500mg
Rutin 50mg
Digestive Enzymes
Probiotics: Acidopholus, Bifidus, Bulgaricus
Green Cruciferous Vegetables
Herbs: Siberian Ginseng, Alfalfa, Red Clover
Bee Pollen
Barley Grass
Chlorella
Green Tea
Rooibos Tea

KEY TO THE LISTINGS

**1000 micrograms (mcg) =
1 milligram (mg)**

**1000 milligrams (mg) =
1 gram (gm)**

**1000 grams (gm) =
1 kilo**

IU = International Units

MDA: Minimum Daily Allowance
= The amount of a nutrient that the
Federal Drug Administration (FDA)
says is required to maintain bodily
health.

RDA: Recommended Daily
Allowance = The amount of a
nutrient that the FDA recommends
be taken daily.

THERAPEUTIC DOSE: The
amount of nutrient that health
professionals prescribe for certain
medical conditions, and that must be
administered under their care.

Items within an entry in **bold type**
have their own entries on the list.

THE DICTIONARY

1-AD (1-androstene-3 beta, 17 beta diol) is a hormone that converts to 1 testosterone, which is seven times as anabolic as testosterone. It does not transform into an estrogen, thereby reducing water retention and secondary sexual feminine characteristics in men. (182)

5-HTP (L-5-hydroxy-tryptophan) is derived from griffonia (griffonia simplicifolia) seeds, and is the immediate precursor to serotonin, the brain nutrient for relaxation. It is effective in treating insomnia, fibromyalgia, depression, binge-eating, weight loss, and chronic headaches. It can be used in place of the FDA-banned l-**tryptophan** to increase serotonin levels in the brain.

7-keto DHEA (3-acetyl-7-oxo-dehydroepiandrosterone) is a naturally-occurring metabolite derived from **DHEA**, but is more potent than that hormone, and cannot be converted to active androgens (testosterone) and estrogens. It is used to strengthen the immune system, and to enhance memory. It activates various thermogenic enzymes, and has weight loss and anti-aging properties. (182)

acerola is a fruit from the West Indies that is high in **Vitamin C**, and is a good free-radical scavenger. It is useful against colds, flu, viral hepatitis and poliomyelitis. It can be used in high dosages safely.

acetyl l-carnitine is an amino acid complex used to treat Alzheimer's disease, depression, and cerebrovascular insufficiency. It increases the activity of the neurotransmitters acetylcholine and dopamine. It is an antioxidant, and reduces the formation of lipofuscin, the aging pigment found in the heart, nerve cells and skin. It has a major effect on short-term memory, and it affects major depression and changes in circadian hormonal rhythms, similar to **melatonin**. A pregnant or nursing woman should not take it. The usual dose is 500 to 2000mg. (188)

acidophilus is lactic bacteria that are one-celled micro-organisms essential in the digestive tract for performing many functions necessary to promote immunity and proper nutrition. It helps digestion, produces natural antibiotics, manufactures vital nutrients, and regulates elimination. Acidophilus also balances digestion, and is a treatment for diarrhea and constipation. It is available as powder, tablets, capsules or liquid, and should be refrigerated when purchased and stored.

alanine (L-Alanine) is an amino acid involved in the metabolism of glucose, and is recommended for hypoglycemia.

Albion process see **chelated minerals**

alfalfa is high in **Vitamin K** and other vitamins, **iron**, and numerous trace minerals. It is an estrogen precursor useful in menopause, an aid in treating arthritis, and is a mild diuretic and anti-inflammatory.

alginates are found in all brown seaweeds and are available as a gel. They are a rich source of many minerals, and act as an aid to detoxification.

alkylglycerols see **shark liver oil**

allantoin see **aloe vera**

allicin is found in garlic, and is anti-microbial against viruses, bacteria and fungus. It detoxifies cancerous chemicals, lowers cholesterol, enhances immunity, and helps to treat arthritic and rheumatoid conditions.

aloe vera is high in allantoin, a natural healing substance that stimulates cell regeneration. Its historical use is for burns, ulcers, hemorrhoids and constipation. It contains enzymes that break down

dead cells and ope[...]
aids in pain relief an[...]
healing. Aloe vera ha[...]
anti-fungal and anti-ba[...]
properties, and is used b[...]
AIDS patients.

alpha hydroxy acids loosen the
bond between the top layers of dead
skin cells. This loosening stimulates
a natural sloughing-off process of the
dead cells, allowing new skin cells to
emerge, thereby reducing wrinkles
and sun damage.

alpha ketoglutarate (AKG) is an
amino acid important in the Krebs
Cycle (production of energy in the
cells). It increases stamina, recovery
time, energy, and aids in the removal
of waste by-products such as
ammonia and lactic acid build-up in
the muscles. It appears to improve
mental clarity and physical
performance. (177)

alpha-lipoic acid is an antioxidant
which moves easily through the
cells. It recycles both **Vitamin E**
and **Vitamin C** in the body. It has
been used for the detoxification of
heavy metal poisoning, and in the
treatment of atherosclerosis,
diabetes, stress, and cataracts.
Recent research indicates that lipoic
acid prevents HIV replication. It has
the ability to protect DNA in the cell
nucleus, and to bolster cellular

35

...one levels, which protect the
...s from oxidation.

amino acids are the building blocks
of protein. They form the muscles,
tendons, ligaments, organs, glands,
hair, nails, and vital body fluids.
They are necessary for the growth
and maintenance of the body, and a
necessary component of the lymph,
blood, enzymes, antibodies,
neurotransmitters, and chromosomes.
(17)

amla is a rejuvenator, and is
considered the richest source of
Vitamin C found in nature. It is
drawn from an Indian gooseberry
which can contain more than
1000mg of natural **Vitamin C**.

amylase is an enzyme that digests
sugar, starches, fats, carbohydrates
and dead white blood cells. It aids in
the control of LDL (bad) cholesterol,
and is helpful in lowering high levels
of triglycerides in the blood. It is
involved in anti-inflammatory
reactions, and helps protect against
abscesses, psoriasis, eczema, hives,
allergic reactions to bee stings,
asthma, emphysema, and all types of
herpes.

andrographis (chuanxinlian,
kalmegh) is an herb used historically
for colds, flu, digestion, malaria,
hepatitis and snakebite. It enhances
immunity and liver function, lowers

blood sugar, and strengthens the heart.

androstenedione is a natural hormone produced by the adrenal gland. In the body, it converts to testosterone, which increases muscle mass, enhances sexual desire, and elevates mood. It should be used with caution.

androsterone is a steroid hormone, excreted in the urine, that reinforces masculine characteristics. It should not be taken by men under the age of eighteen, and women should use it with caution.

angelica root (angelica archangelica) is an anti-spasmodic that is a treatment for strong menstrual cramps with scanty flow, intestinal colic, and poor digestion. It is also an expectorant for coughs.

anise seed (pimpinella anisum) eases indigestion, flatulence and colic. It is also an anti-spasmodic and expectorant.

antioxidants are nutrients that donate an electron to a free-radical and thereby neutralize it. (23)

apple cider vinegar adjusts the pH of the system, and aids the growth of **acidophilus** in the intestines. It is acidic from acetic and malic acids, a good source of **potassium** and enzymes. It improves digestion, and has antibody-like properties. It acts as a blood-cleanser, flushing out the vascular system and thinning out cholesterol in the blood.

arginine (L-Arginine) is an amino acid which is a prime stimulant of growth hormone release, increasing muscle tone and decreasing fat. It aids in liver and ammonia detoxification, promotes a healthy immune system, and blocks the formation of tumors. It increases sperm count and motility, reduces appetite, and aids in fat metabolism. It should be avoided by anyone with the herpes virus, schizophrenia, and by women who are pregnant or lactating. (179,189)

arnica (arnica montana) is an herb prepared homeopathically, used topically over unbroken skin, for sprains, swelling, bruises and strains.

aroma therapy uses the therapeutic characteristics of aromatic essential oils. These oils tend to work very quickly to aid the body's natural defenses, and to balance the body's systems. (170)

artichoke is a vegetable that aids digestion, reduces cholesterol, and strengthens the liver. It contains cynarin and scolymoside, which stimulate bile secretion while lowering cholesterol and triglyceride levels. It has some diuretic properties that aid in the elimination of protein in the urine through the kidneys.

ascorbic acid see **Vitamin C**

ascorbyl palmitate see **C ester**, **ester C**, **Vitamin C**

ashwagandha (winter cherry, Indian ginseng, withnia somnifera) is an Ayurvedic herb that has adaptogenic properties similar to Chinese **ginseng**, and has traditionally been used as an aphrodisiac, and for rejuvenating muscle tissues and sexual fluids. It is also used to treat chronic exhaustion.

asparagine (L-Asparagine) is an amino acid that nourishes the central nervous system and enhances emotional stability. It helps the liver process the transformation of amino acids into proteins.

aspartic acid (L-Aspartic acid) is an amino acid that works with **calcium** and **magnesium** to support the cardiovascular system. It aids in the removal of ammonia, and is a precursor to **threonine**, which increases stamina and reduces fatigue. It is used clinically for depression and for protecting the liver. It aids the immune system's production of antibodies and immunoglobulins.

astaxanthin is a pinkish-red carotenoid that is a very potent antioxidant. It helps to recycle **Vitamin E**, **beta carotene**, **lycopene** and **glutathione** in the body.

astragalus (huang qi) is an immune-system tonic used for colds and flu. It reduces fatigue, but is not recommended for a fever. It aids digestion, and is used to treat weak lungs, cancer and tumors. (189)

avena sativa see **oatseed**

Bach flower essences are thirty-eight flower essences discovered by Dr. Edward Bach, and used to treat emotional conditions within a person. (165)

B-Complex Vitamins (see individual listings) **Vitamin B1** (thiamine), **Vitamin B2** (riboflavin), **Vitamin B3** (niacin), **Vitamin B5** (pantothenic acid), **Vitamin B6** (pyridoxine), **Vitamin B12** (cobalamin), **biotin**, choline, inositol, **PABA** (para aminobenzoic acid), and **folic acid** (folate). (189,198)

balm of gilead (populus spp.) soothes, disinfects, and is an astringent for mucous membranes. It is an expectorant, and is used to treat laryngitis, coughs and sore throat.

barberry root (berberis fe...
a digestive and appetite stimula...
and stimulates bile flow and liver
function. It helps reduce fevers, and
is an antiseptic and anti-convulsant.

barley green has a high
chlorophyll content, and contains
trace minerals, enzymes and **beta
carotene**. It helps to regulate bowel
function, and provides antioxidant
support. It can significantly decrease
the symptoms of jet-lag, and is a
good source of **SOD** (superoxide
dismutase). (201)

bayberry bark (myrica cerifera) is
an astringent used for bleeding gums,
sore throat, diarrhea, intestinal
inflammation, and post-partum
hemorrhage. It is also a vasodilator
of skin and mucous membranes.

bee pollen is a nourishing and
energizing 'super food' which
contains **B-Complex** vitamins, trace
minerals, proteins, carbohydrates,
fats and enzymes, as well as
numerous other nutritional elements.
Bee pollen provides energy,
enhances mental and physical
performance, and aids menstrual and
prostate problems. (177,201)

beet root (beta vulgaris) is rich in
iron, and aids the liver and spleen.

bentonite clay can be used as a
poultice or facial mask to cleanse the

...rnally as a
...anser.

... (see **Vitamin A**) is
... two molecules which
... ...ed in the liver to **Vitamin
A**, ...s use requires a healthy
liver. It is a very powerful
antioxidant. The RDA is 4,000 to
5,000IU. The usual dose is
25,000IU daily. Beta carotene is
converted to **Vitamin A** only
according to the body's needs, and is
therefore non-toxic.

beta-1,3-glucan (from barley or
oats) is a source of soluble dietary
fiber that aids in the reduction of
cholesterol. It is rich in **tocotrienols**,
which are very strong antioxidants,
and is obtained from purified yeast,
with much research reporting it able
to stimulate non-specific immunity.
Glucan is the most widely and
commonly observed macrophage
activator in nature. It reduces
cholesterol, and has a broad,
enhancing effect on the immune
system. (189)

betaine (trimethylglycine) is an
important digestive and liver
lipotropic substance. Betaine
stimulates bile production, and
converts protein metabolites such as
homocysteine into **glutamine** and
other energy components.

42

beta sitosterol is a vegetable phytosterol that lowers serum cholesterol and reduces carcinogens in the colon.

bioperine is an extract of black pepper that aids digestion and the absorption of nutrients. (see **peperine**)

BHT (butylated hydroxytoluene) is an FDA-approved preservative for oils, food, and fats. It is a powerful antioxidant, and is an effective aid against the herpes virus.

bifidus (bifidobacterium) is a friendly bacteria that resides in the large intestine. Its presence discourages harmful bacteria, and fungi such as candida, from living there, and helps the large intestine dispose of unused food. It also produces **B-Complex** vitamins, enzymes, and lactic acid that help the body complete the digestive process.

bilberry is an antiseptic and astringent. It enhances eye health, and helps prevent macular degeneration. It is used successfully as a mouthwash, for treating diarrhea, and for reducing varicose veins. It also strengthens connective tissue. Its use can interfere with **iron** absorption.

biloba see **ginkgo**

e a family of
consist of thousands
its and active
at provide a variety of
rus bioflavonoids help
strength of the
capilla , which can correct
excessive cell permeability. Signs of
deficiency include the tendency to
bruise and bleed easily. There are
many other bioflavonoids that have
other specific benefits.

biotin (d-biotin) is a **B-Complex**
vitamin necessary for healthy hair,
skin and nails. It is important in the
metabolism of essential fatty acids,
sugar, and proteins. Biotin improves
immune response and glucose
tolerance in diabetics. The fungus
candida in the intestine will not
multiply where biotin is present.
Biotin, along with other **B-Complex**
vitamins, benefits hair loss, dandruff,
scalp problems, eczema, and
dermatitis. Biotin has no RDA, but
in 1980 the National Research
Council has set a range of 100 to
200mcg daily. The recommended
daily dose is 600mcg. Therapeutic
dosage ranges from 1000 to
3000mcg for hair, nails and scalp,
and up to 9mg per day for diabetics.
Eating raw egg whites can block the
absorption of biotin.

Biotron process see **chelated
minerals**

black cherry has been successful in the treatment of gout and arthritis. Some markets are mixing black cherries with hamburger to reduce cholesterol and uric acid in people who consume red meat.

black cohosh is used for menstrual cramping and for relief from hot flashes in menopausal women. It is a mild sedative, and is a treatment for spasms. It is beneficial to the heart and circulation, and can reduce cholesterol levels. It should not be used during pregnancy, but aids in inducing labor and childbirth.

black currant oil includes d-gamma linoleic acid (**GLA**), alpha linoleic acid (ALA) an **omega 3** oil, and a balanced group of essential fatty acids. It is an anti-inflammatory, and is useful for PMS, skin problems, and diabetes. It is a potent antioxidant.

black walnut (juglans nigra) is an anti-fungal herb used to promote bowel regularity, fight fungal infections, and dispel parasites.

blessed thistle (cnicus benedictus) increases lactation, and is a treatment for indigestion, chronic headaches, diarrhea and hemorrhage.

blue cohosh (caulophyllum thalictroides) is a uterine tonic and a diuretic, anti-spasmodic, and mild expectorant. It should be used in the last trimester of pregnancy only.

blue flag root (iris versicolor) is a liver purgative, blood purifier, cathartic and diuretic. It is used for constipation, biliousness, and eruptive skin conditions. Use in low doses only.

blue green algae (aphanizemenon flos-aqua) a phytoplankton that is a potent brain food, and an excellent source of micro-nutrients which increase cognitive and physical efficiency. It is easily digested, readily absorbed, and rich in **chlorophyll**, proteins, nucleic acids, nitrogen compounds and other essential nutrients, including **Vitamin B12**.

blue vervain (verbena hastata) soothes cranky children, is a sedative, an anti-depressant and anti-spasmodic, and is used as a mild analgesic.

boldo promotes fat digestion by stimulating the secretion of bile, and helps to neutralize excess stomach acid. It is used to treat liver, gall bladder and bowel dysfunctions. Other reputed uses are for urogenital inflammations, gout, hepatitis, rheumatism, and as an antiseptic.

boneset (eupatorium perfoliatum) is used for flu symptoms, aches and pains, and helps clear mucous congestion. It reduces fevers and the pain of muscular rheumatism.

borage oil (see **GLA**) is a gland balancer and adrenal tonic helpful for diabetes, PMS, and skin problems. It also aids cardiovascular function, and contains essential fatty acids such as d-gamma linoleic acid. (224)

boron is a trace mineral that affects **calcium**, **magnesium** and **phosphorous** metabolism. Boron increases estrogen production in menopausal women. It also converts **Vitamin D** into its most active form. Boron has shown to be very beneficial for people suffering from joint problems, and as an aid in reducing bone loss. The usual dose is 3mg daily. Excessive use of boron can be toxic.

boswellia is an Ayurvedic herb used to reduce the pain and inflammation of arthritic conditions.

bovine cartilage (tracheal cartilage) has anti-inflammatory properties. It provides components that the body utilizes in synthesizing cartilage. It is non-toxic, and is a powerful agent that provides relief to sufferers of osteo-arthritis and rheumatoid arthritis. It has also been used by people suffering from heart conditions, cancer, and severe skin allergies. It is a biological response modifier, that activates the immune system when conditions require it, or suppresses it in rheumatoid conditions.

brewers yeast (nutritional yeast) is a rich source of **inositol, choline,** most of the other **B-Complex** vitamins, trace minerals, amino acids, and ribo-nucleic acid (**RNA**). Different strains of yeast have different nutritional profiles. Yeast is recommended for skin problems, anorexia, high cholesterol, anemia, and for improving vision and increasing energy.

broccoli is a rich source of **DIM,** and contains sulforaphane, an aid in detoxification.

bromelain is an enzyme from pineapple that aids in the digestion of protein. It is an effective anti-inflammatory if taken on an empty stomach, and is useful for reducing bruising, and healing wounds. It inhibits blood clotting without the occurrence of excessive bleeding.

bulgaricus (i.b. bulgaricum) is the friendly bacteria used in the production of yogurt. It is an excellent detoxifier that greatly aids in the elimination of toxins through the bowels. It helps relieve stress on the liver, and is very helpful for those with hepatitis C. (190)

burdock root (arctium lappa) is a blood cleanser and anti-microbial, and is used for skin eruptions, dry, scaly skin conditions, and certain cancers. It is also a digestive stimulant, and lowers blood sugar.

butcher's broom is an herb containing ruscogenins which reduces hemorrhoids, varicose veins, and anal itching. It aids 'heavy legs,' a circulatory problem of the veins in the legs. It constricts the veins, and reduces their permeability and fragility. It is also an anti-inflammatory.

butterbur (petasites hybridus) is a muscle relaxant, and is used to treat intestinal colic, asthma, migraine, and painful menses.

calcium is the most abundant mineral in the body. It is vital for healthy bones and teeth, with 99% of the body's calcium found in the skeleton. Calcium is necessary for a regular heartbeat, muscular contraction, clotting of blood, and the transmission of nerve impulses. The bone meal form contains protein, calcium, and **phospohorus**. Dolomite is a carbonate form, with **magnesium** and other trace minerals. The carbonate form is poorly absorbed compared to the citrate form. The aspartate and orotate forms are considered the most therapeutic because of their very high level of assimilation. The most important caveat for calcium is to be certain to include other minerals, especially **magnesium**. A good rule of thumb is to take half as much **magnesium** as you do calcium. Too much calcium can result in an imbalance, with the body laying calcium down in soft tissue resulting in various disease conditions, including premature aging from free-radical damage, and from calcification, leading to arthritis. The RDA for adults is 800 to 1200mg. It is possible to maintain calcium balance even at very low intakes of 200 to 400mg daily. (15)

calcium hydroxyl apetite is a very absorbable form of **calcium** derived from cattle that are free-range and organically fed.

calendula is used to reduce pain, and aid healing. It is especially helpful for joint inflammation, and is used topically for wounds, ulcers, abscesses and burns. It is a treatment for diaper rash, and for reducing fevers.

California poppy is a sedative herb useful as an aid for sleep and hyperactivity.

caprylic acid is a short-chain fatty acid which helps maintain proper bacterial balance in the intestines. It is also used to combat fungus, especially candida.

carnitine (L-Carnitine) is a pseudo-amino acid with vitamin status (Vitamin Bt). It helps regulate fat metabolism and lowers cholesterol and triglyceride levels. It is very important for the heart, where it prevents fatty build-up. It also prevents the build-up of ketones (fat waste-products) in the blood, and aids in weight loss. Another form, **Acetyl-L-Carnitine** (see separate listing) plays a key role in maintaining normal brain and nerve functions in the elderly. It is also an excellent antioxidant, and increases cerebral blood flow. It improves short-term memory and depression, and stabilizes circadian hormonal rhythms, similar to **melatonin**. (180,197)

carnosine is an amino acid made from **histidine** and **alanine**. It is a potent antioxidant that protects the membranes of cells, improves heart function, and aids in wound healing. It removes (**chelates**) heavy metals from the body, acts as a neurotransmitter, and protects against peptic ulcers. It is a marker of aging that protects proteins from destruction.

carrageenan is a water-soluble gum in gel form prepared from red seaweed. It is an aid in detoxification.

cascara sagrada bark (rhamnus purshiana) is a laxative, mild liver stimulant, and bitter tonic.

catalase is an **enzyme** that clears toxins, radiation, free-radicals, infections, and other poisonous wastes. It adds energy to the body and clarity to the mind.

catnip (nepeta cataria) is used for indigestion, flatulence and colic. It is a mild astringent, and a specific for childhood diarrhea.

cat's claw (una de gato) is a treatment for ulcers, arthritis, and immune-system dysfunction. It enhances white blood-cell activity, and cleanses the intestinal tract. However, it is not to be used during pregnancy.

cayenne (capsicum spp.) equalizes circulation for cold hands and feet, strengthens the heart, has stimulant and antiseptic properties, and is used as gargle for persistent cough.

CCK (cholecystokinin) is one of the major regulating hormones that controls digestion. It helps the gall bladder to empty, and the pancreas to produce pancreatic enzymes. It is also used as an aid for weight reduction.

CDP choline (cytidine 5'-diphoscholine) is a water-soluble compound necessary for the synthesis of **phosphatidyl choline**, the major constituent of the brain. It aids brain metabolism by helping synthesize acetylcholine, and easily passes through the blood-brain barrier directly into the nervous system. It helps protect the brain, aids in its recovery from injuries, and reduces edema caused by stroke.

cedar berry (thuja spp.) is an astringent and expectorant. It has been used to decrease the need for insulin therapy.

cell salts (tissue-cell salts) were discovered by William Schuessler. It appears that every form of illness has an imbalance of one or more of these mineral salts. They are prepared homeopathically, and are used to stimulate normal metabolism and restore health. (163)

C ester (ascorbyl palmitate) (see **ester C, Vitamin C**) is the fat-soluble form of **Vitamin C**, which can be stored in the body and organs. It is frequently used in anti-wrinkle skin products.

chamomile is gentle and effective for children as a sedative, and for reducing fevers. It improves the health of the gums and skin, and is a digestive aid and appetite stimulant.

53

It should be used intermittently to avoid triggering a ragweed allergy.

charcoal is nature's detoxifier, and is used to absorb poisons. It helps alleviate gas, bloating, food poisoning, and diarrhea.

chaste berry (vitex agnus-castrus, chaste tree) stimulates and normalizes pituitary function, and is used for PMS, menstrual cramps, and menopause problems.

chelation formulas are used to remove heavy metals from the body. The most common one is **EDTA**, which also removes excess **calcium**.

chelated minerals are mineral molecules surrounded by an amino acid molecule, or with some other organic molecule, making them more easily absorbed from the digestive tract, and from there into the bloodstream. Two excellent processes used to create chelated minerals are the Albion process, and the Biotron process. Price is a very good indicator of quality in chelated minerals. The more chelating material present, the better the absorption, and the more it costs.

chickweed (stellaria media) is a diuretic and thyroid regulator. It increases cell-membrane permeability, and helps to emulsify

and mobilize fat cells. It is high in
lecithin.

chitosan (chitosol, 'fat-blocker') is
primarily used as an aid in weight
loss and in the lowering of
cholesterol. It is produced from the
skeletons of shellfish, and its
function is to absorb fat molecules in
the stomach, and then to eliminate
them in the feces without being
digested.

chlorella is a single-cell **blue-green
algae** which is higher in **chlorophyll**
than any other plant. It contains a
unique combination of molecules
called Controlled Growth Factor
(CGF) that improves energy and
strengthens the immune system. It is
an excellent detoxifier of heavy
metals and is a complete protein
which contains high amounts of
Vitamin B12, the essential fatty acid
gamma linoleic acid (**GLA**), other
vitamins, minerals, enzymes and
fiber. It strengthens the liver,
detoxifies the colon, helps maintain
proper weight and muscle tone, and
enhances digestion and immunity. It
is beneficial for MS, radiation
damage protection, and chronic
fatigue syndrome. (200)

chlorophyll is the green pigment in
plants that produces oxygen through
photosynthesis, and has been used in
place of blood for transfusions.
(Chlorophyll has a **magnesium**

molecule, as compared to blood which has an **iron** molecule.) It is effective against infections, sinusitis, gum disease, and skin conditions. It is a natural internal deodorant, and an aid against halitosis, kidney stones, and is helpful during menstruation. It is useful against many cancers. Its most active ingredient is chlorophyllin

choline (choline bitartrate, choline chloride, phosphatidylcholine) is essential in making the important neurotransmitter acetylcholine. It is necessary for the proper metabolism of fats, especially in the liver, and is essential for the formation of the cell membranes. It also acts as a lubricant in the linings of the lungs and arteries. Choline has the ability to reduce fatty infiltration of the liver, and offers great benefits in the treatment of liver disorders and in lowering cholesterol. It is an immune-system stimulant able to inhibit the development of certain types of tumors. Choline has a RDA of 9mg. The suggested daily dose is 200 to 500mg. The therapeutic dose is from 5,000 to as high as 30,000mg. Choline is non-toxic; however, it can be metabolized in the intestines by bacteria-forming trimethylamine, which produces a fishy odor. It is recommended to take **chlorophyll** and **acidophilus** supplements to help reduce this effect when taking high doses.

chondroitin sulfate (CSA) is produced from **bovine cartilage**. It acts as an anti-inflammatory agent which is helpful to the joints, the heart, and the immune system.

chromium is an essential trace mineral. It is the primary component of the biologically-active Glucose Tolerance Factor (GTF), a combination of **chromium**, niacin (Vitamin B3), and **glutathione** which boosts the action of insulin, and therefore helps to reduce sugar cravings, which aids in the control of diabetes and hypoglycemia. It reduces high levels of cholesterol and triglycerides in the blood stream. Chromium helps build healthy arteries, converts fat to muscle, curbs the appetite, and raises body metabolism. The usual dose is 50 to 200mcg daily. The therapeutic dose is 400 to 600mcg daily. Trivalent chromium, the form found in most chromium supplements, is documented to be extremely safe. Another safe form is picolinate. (180,203)

chrysin is an **isoflavone** from passiflora coerulea that increases testosterone in athletes, and blocks its conversion into estrogen.

chymotrypism is a proteolytic enzyme.

Citrimax (citrin) is the trade name for the standardized extract of garcinia cambogia fruit (Indian berry). The active ingredient is a compound of hydroxycitric acid (HCA). It aids in weight loss by reducing appetite, increasing metabolism, and inhibiting fatty-acid synthesis in the liver.

citrulline (L-Citrulline) is an amino acid that detoxifies ammonia from cells and promotes energy.

ciwujuia root is a Chinese herb that reduces the build-up of lactic acid in the muscles, increases the metabolism of fats rather than carbohydrates for energy, and aids the immune system. Athletes use it to improve performance and recovery.

CLA (conjugated linoleic acid) is a fatty acid that blocks the effects of muscle-wasting stress hormones such as cortisol, regulates protein metabolism, and helps prevent hardening of the arteries. It is an aid in weight loss, and in the proper burning of fat. The usual dosage is 600 to 1200mg per day.

cleavers (gallium aparine) is a lymphatic tonic and diuretic used for swollen glands, cystitis, ulcers, tumors, skin disorders, and painful urination.

CMO (cetyl myristoleate) is a fatty acid that acts as a modulator for the immune system, and as a lubricant for joints. It shows promise as an arthritic protective factor, and in possibly relieving the symptoms of arthritis.

cobalamin see **Vitamin B12**

cod liver oil see **fish oils**

collagen is the fibrous protein matrix which provides support for the body in the form of cartilage, bones, and connective tissue. **Vitamin C**, **lysine**, **proline** and **silica** are necessary for collagen formation. It is the glue of the body.

colloidal minerals are minerals in a liquid suspension, and are the most easily absorbed in the body. Avoid inorganic formulas, and look for products derived from sea vegetables, which are free of pollutants.

colloidal silver is pure metallic ionic silver held in liquid suspension by an electrical charge. It is a potent antibiotic that disables an enzyme used by bacteria, fungi and viruses for metabolism, which do not appear to develop an immunity to it; it is non-toxic in the body. Formulas range from 5 to 500ppm (parts per million).

colostrum promotes balance in the immune system. It contains the full spectrum of all immunoglobulins, which contain thousands of different specific antibodies. Colostrum treats auto-immune diseases by establishing a correct ratio between T-helper cells and T-killer cells, so that immunity remains strong, but not destructive. Colostrum is also high in growth hormones that increase body weight through muscle growth. (190)

coltsfoot (tussilago farfara) is a soothing expectorant, and is used as an anti-spasmodic, anti-inflammatory, and astringent. It is also used to treat irritating coughs, bronchitis, asthma, laryngitis, throat catarrh, and for sores and ulcers.

comfrey leaf (symphytum officinalis) speeds healing of sprains, strains, fractures and surface wounds. It is a good source of the natural healer, **allantoin**.

copper is needed for the absorption and control of **iron**, and in the formation of red blood cells. It is important for bone formation, immune function, and oxidative enzymes which destroy toxins in the liver and bloodstream. Copper is necessary for the production of **SOD** (superoxide dismutase) which protects cell membranes from the attack of free-radicals, for proper skin and hair pigmentation, and for the protection of nerve fibers. Copper is best in the **chelated** form. It is usually found in supplements in the form of copper sabacate. The general requirements for copper for an adult is 1.5 to 3mg daily. High dosages of copper, though rare, can be toxic. Copper needs to be balanced with at least 22mg of **zinc**. The usual dose of copper is 2mg.

CoQ-10 is an important vitamin-like nutrient. It is an enzyme that helps produce energy in the cells, and is a potent antioxidant. It is used clinically, especially in Japan, for heart disease, high blood pressure, immune-system stimulation, slowing the aging process, periodontal disease, peptic ulcers, muscular dystrophy, and heart disease. There is evidence that it can increase the volume of oxygen in the blood by as much as fifteen percent. (190,205)

cordyceps is a fungus that strengthens the immune system, protects the lungs, and increases oxygen in the body. It is also a strong antioxidant.

coriander seed (coriandrum sativum) eases intestinal grippe and diarrhea, especially in children. It is an appetite stimulant, and increases the secretion of digestive juices.

coriolus (coriolus versicolor, turkey tail) is a mushroom extract which is a potent enhancer of the immune system. It is an aid to certain cancer therapies, and protects white blood cells from chemotherapy damage.

corn silk (zea mays) is a soothing diuretic, and is used for renal and urinary irritation, bedwetting, cystitis, urethritis, and prostatitis.

couch grass (agropyron repens) is an anti-microbial used to treat cystitis, urethritis, prostatitis, and for kidney stones and gravel.

cow parsnip root (heracleum lanatum) is an anti-nauseant and anti-spasmodic, and is an analgesic for sore teeth and gums.

cramp bark (viburnum opulus) relaxes muscle tension and spasms, and treats ovarian pain and uterine cramps. It is also used to prevent a threatened miscarriage.

cranberry is a diuretic and urinary antiseptic that is excellent for bladder and kidney infections. It acidifies the urine and prevents bacteria from attaching to the walls of the bladder. It is best to buy the concentrate without sugar for drinking, and it is also available in capsules.

creatine (creatine monohydrate) is an amino acid that can enhance expended cellular energy without the need for carbohydrates, fats, or oxygen to recharge the muscles. It is a source of quick energy, buffers lactic acid buildup, and reduces exercise fatigue. It is used extensively by athletes and body-builders. (181,205)

cryptoxanthin is a potent carotenoid which is a strong antioxidant, and protects against cervical cancer in women.

culvers root (leptandra virginica) is an herb that acts as a mild laxative by stimulating the liver, thereby releasing bile.

curcumin is derived from the herb, **turmeric**. It is a potent antioxidant that helps protect against heart disease and many cancers. It also reduces inflammation in rheumatoid arthritis, and prevents blood clots. It reduces candida in the gut by eliminating **iron** from the colon.

cysteine (L-Cysteine) is a sulfur-bearing amino acid that aids in skin formation and detoxification. Cysteine is the major component of hair, nails and skin, and protects the liver and brain from harmful toxins and free-radical damage. It is a precursor to **glutathione**, which also neutralizes harmful toxins in the liver and brain. L-Cysteine requires the presence of **Vitamin C** in a one to three ratio for safe utilization.

daidzen see **soy supplements**
damiana (tunera aphrodisiaca) is a tonic herb used to aid the central nervous system, reduce anxiety and enhance sexual desire and performance.

dandelion (taraxacum off.) is a mild laxative, blood cleanser, and a powerful and safe diuretic. It is used for inflammation and congestion of the liver and gall bladder, and for obstructive jaundice.

deer antler velvet is a source of lipids, proteins, prostaglandins, **glucosamine**, **chondroitin** sulfate A, and antibiotic-like substances. It is a tonic for the reproductive and circulatory systems, has anti-cancer properties, and improves athletic strength and performance. It aids arthritic conditions, mental function, and the heart. It reduces stress, inhibits PMS and impotence, and lowers the risk of stroke and heart attack.

devil's club (oplopanax horridum) is a pancreatic tonic, blood sugar regulator, and increases endurance.

DGL (deglycyrrhizinated licorice) is a safe form of licorice that helps soothe ulcers. It reduces pain from arthritis without the glycyrrhetinic acid that can raise blood pressure.

DHA see **fish oils**

DHEA (dehydroepiandrosterone) is naturally produced by the adrenal glands, and is the most abundant hormone in the human body, but its levels diminish with age. It can be converted into estrogen and testosterone. DHEA improves immune function, lowers the risk of heart disease, and enhances mood, memory, and REM sleep. It aids in proper weight maintenance, and may be helpful against cancer, HIV, and lupus. Only a few living creatures, specifically humans and other closely related primates, produce DHEA. Studies show that men with the highest DHEA levels retain better functioning into their later years. DHEA may inhibit tumor growth in pre-menopausal women, but stimulate the growth of breast cancer in post-menopausal women. DHEA supplements should not be taken if there is any indication of liver cancer, or a family history of hormone-related cancers such as those of the breast or prostate gland. DHEA has been used as a treatment for some forms of psychiatric disorders, including schizophrenia. (190)

digestive enzymes see **enzymes**

dill (anethum graveolens) is used for flatulence and colic, especially in children, and stimulates lactation.

DIM (di-indolyl methane) is made from cruciferous vegetables such as broccoli and Brussels sprouts. It aids in the breakdown of estrogen into beneficial, or 'good' estrogen metabolites (known as 2-hydroxy estrogens). These help to protect the heart and brain with their antioxidant activity. At the same time, DIM reduces the levels of 'bad' estrogen metabolites (produced by environmental toxins and obesity, and known as 16-hydroxy estrogens), which can cause unwanted weight gain, and breast, uterine and prostate cancers. DIM is highly recommended for women on HRT (Hormone Replacement Therapy), or who are at risk for breast cancer.

DLPA (dl-phenylalanine) is a combination of the D and L forms of **phenylalanine**. which is a powerful painkiller, and which does not incorporate into the body's proteins. It is especially good for chronic pain, such as from arthritis, migraine or menstruation. The D form is very expensive, and is usually combined with the L form as DL-Phenylalanine in a one-to-one ratio. Pregnant women, people with high blood pressure, those suffering from phenylketonuria (PKU), pigmented melanoma skin cancer, anxiety attacks, or diabetes should not take either form.

DMAE (dimethylaminoethanol) is a natural amino alcohol, and a precursor to **choline** and acetylcholine in the brain. DMAE is reported to elevate mood, increase intelligence, improve memory and learning, and extend lifespan. It is used topically to reduce wrinkles. It is transported directly across the blood-brain barrier. DMAE supplementation is best started with a small amount, and increased gradually at weekly intervals to avoid a possible temporary condition of muscle stiffness in the neck and shoulders.

DMG (n,n-dimethylglycine, Vitamin B15) is useful in the production of neurotransmitters, hormones, DNA, **choline**, and **methionine**. It enhances the immune system, normalizes blood glucose levels, and reduces high blood pressure. It improves oxygen utilization, reduces lactic acid formation, and aids in cell detoxification. It also improves liver, pancreas, and adrenal function, and enhances athletic performance. DMG is excellent for increasing endurance, sharpening vision, and halting allergy reactions and headaches in their early stages. (175,205)

DMSO (dimethylsulfoxide) is by-product of the paper industry, and is an excellent solvent. It is used only topically, produces a fishy, garlic-like taste, and is easily absorbed through the skin and blood vessels. It carries anything else on the surface of the skin inside the body with it. It reduces pain from injuries, and is used for sprains, arthritis, and sciatica. It is beneficial for headaches, herpes, and skin problems. It should be used with great care on clean skin only.

dolomite is a natural form of **magnesium** carbonate, **calcium** carbonate, and other trace minerals. It is used to combat bone loss.

dong quai is a female hormone regulator known by some as 'female **ginseng**'. It is used for cramping, PMS and menopause. It is a mild sedative and thins the blood. Therefore, it should be taken with medical advice if one is taking anti-coagulants, or is having a bleeding problem.

ecdysterone is a plant or insect extract that increases nitrogen retention and protein synthesis. It stimulates metabolism and improves nerve and muscular function. It is anabolic, and requires the addition of extra protein in the diet to be most effective. The usual dose for bodybuilders is from 80 to

600mg per day, on a six-week cycle. (183)

echinacea is a powerful immune-system stimulant used for colds, flu, infections and allergies. It is an anti-viral and anti-bacterial agent. It also strengthens the lymphatic system. (191)

EDTA is a chemical that aids in the removal of heavy metals and excessive **calcium** within the soft tissues of the body.

egg yolk lecithin is a fluidizer of the cell membranes. As cells age, the membranes become stiff, and viruses can intrude into the cells. People using egg yolk lecithin have shown a remarkable increase in their ability to fight off infections. It is a rich source of **phosphatidyl choline**.

electrolytes are minerals that support a healthy fluid balance in the cells of the body.

elder flower (sambucus canadensis) is used for upper respiratory infections, colds, flu, hay fever, sinusitis, and fevers. It has anti-catarrhal, diuretic, and expectorant properties.

elderberry extract is both an ancient and modern therapy for colds, flu and fevers. It strengthens cell walls, and inhibits enzymes that weaken the cells.

elecampane root (inula helenium) is an expectorant used for bronchial coughs, bronchitis, emphysema, asthma and bronchial asthma.

enzymes (digestive enzymes, proteolytic enzymes) are catalysts that make metabolism, the chemical reactions necessary for life, possible. They occur naturally in all living things. They digest food, eliminate toxins, and purify the blood. Proteolytic enzymes are taken on an empty stomach, and aid healing, digestion of waste tissue, and reduce bruising. They strengthen the endocrine system, and deliver nutrients and hormones to the cells. They nourish the brain and other organs, balance cholesterol and triglyceride levels, and strengthen the immune system. (183,191,228)

EPA see **fish oils**

ephedra (ma huang) is an herb misunderstood by many people, and is thought of as a stimulant that reduces appetite because of the presence of ephedrine. However, there are many forms of ephedra, and some contain little or no ephedrine. Historically, it is used as a vasodilator for asthma and other respiratory conditions. It is an anti-spasmodic, and stimulates circulation. One form that has little ephedrine is Mormon Tea. If a level of ephedrine is noted on the label, then precautions should be taken. It should not be used by persons with glaucoma, high blood pressure, anxiety attacks, a heart condition, or by someone taking MAO (monoamine oxidase) inhibitors.

essential fatty acids (EFA's) are naturally-occurring unsaturated fats that are considered essential because they are not produced by the human body. The two essential fatty acids are linoleic, sometimes referred to as the omega-6 fatty acid, and alpha-linolenic, referred to as the **omega-3 fatty acid**. Omega-3 and omega-6 fatty acids compete for the same enzymes. A proper balance of these fats in the diet is important for maintenance of good health. The best ratio appears to be 1:1. (191,218,224)

essential oils are highly-concentrated plant extracts that have a unique and specific biochemical composition. They produce potent and particular therapeutic healing properties that are as diverse as the herbs from which they are extracted. (171

Essiac is an herbal formula developed by Renee Caisse, a Canadian nurse, used for detoxification, and to strengthen immunity. It is especially helpful to cancer patients. It contains **burdock root**, sheep sorrel, turkey rhubarb root and **slippery elm bark**.

ester C (see **C ester, Vitamin C**) is a patented formula and a metabolite form of **Vitamin C** that is non-acidic. It is more quickly absorbed and more slowly excreted than regular ascorbic acid, and remains in the system up to twenty-four hours.

evening primrose is high in essential fatty acids, especially d-gamma linoleic acid (see **GLA**). It is used to alleviate PMS, hot flashes, and menstrual problems. It is a mood enhancer, and is used to treat schizophrenia. It reduces high blood pressure, and is helpful for multiple sclerosis, eczema, arthritis, alcoholism, and weight loss. (225)

eyebright (euphrasia officinalis) is an anti-catarrhal, an anti-inflammatory, and an astringent. It is used internally for sinusitis, nasal congestion, and eye inflammations. The leaf infusion is used as an external wash for sore, inflamed eyes.

false unicorn root (chamaelirium luteum) is a reproductive tonic used for delayed menses, ovarian pain, female infertility, and male impotence. It contains estrogen precursors, and, in small doses, eases vomiting in pregnancy. It also helps prevent threatened miscarriage.

fennel seed (foeniculum vulgare) aids digestion and relieves flatulence and colic. It expels mucous, increases lactation, aids weight loss, and is a flavoring agent that increases the digestibility of other herbs.

fenugreek (trigonella foenugraecum) is an anti-inflammatory herb used for digestion, bronchitis, and as an aid in the production and flow of milk in nursing mothers.

feverfew is best known for the relief of migraines with long-term use. It is also used for rheumatoid arthritis, colitis, muscle tension and asthma. Topically, it is useful for insect bites. It also stimulates uterine contractions, and should not be taken during pregnancy.

fiber is divided into soluble fibers of hemicellulose and pectins from bran, oats, legumes and fruit, and insoluble fibers of cellulose from grains. It is very useful for constipation, weight management, lowering cholesterol, protecting the body from cancer, sugar metabolism, and diverticulitis.

figwort (scrophularia spp.) is used internally and topically for eczema.

fish oils (cod liver oil, salmon oil, etc.) (see **omega-3 fatty acids**) provide omega-3 fatty acids that are particularly high in EPA (eicosapentaenoic acid) and DHA (docosahexaenoic acid). These oils lower blood triglycerides and cholesterol, aid circulation, prevent blood clots, and help arthritic conditions. EPA regulates cell hormones, and protects the body from high blood pressure, edema and inflammation. DHA is important for vision, hearing and the reproductive system. (224,225,227)

flavonoids see **bioflavonoids**

flax seed is a bulking agent with nutritive attributes. It is a source of **omega 3** and 6 oils. It also cleanses and lubricates the digestive system, and relieves constipation. It is an aid to inflammation and female disorders. (225)

folate see **folic acid**

folic acid (folate, folacin) has an important role in the synthesis of RNA and DNA. It is essential for proper body growth, fetal development, red blood cell development, the production of brain neurotransmitters, and proper utilization of sugars and amino acids. It helps build antibodies to fight infections, prevents anemia, and functions together with **Vitamin**

B12. Folic acid can reduce homocysteine levels, a condition which thickens the blood and affects cholesterol which can lead to heart disease. Folic acid is a factor in numerous health conditions, from acne to senility. 400mcg is both the usual, and RDA, dose for adults. A daily dose of 800mcg is recommended during pregnancy to guard against spina bifida and other nerve tissue defects. A therapeutic dose of 5 to 10mg is recommended for lesions in the lungs and for cervical dysplasia, and as high as 50mg for depression. **Vitamin B12** should always be included with folic acid supplementation. Folic acid can mask a B12 deficiency that could result in irreparable nerve damage. Many drugs can interfere with folic acid absorption and function, requiring special supplementation considerations from a health professional.

forskolin (coleus forskohlii) is an Ayruvedic herb used for lowering high blood pressure, skin disorders, and strengthening the heart. It appears to prevent glaucoma, stimluate the immune system, and inhibit cancer. This is a powerful herb that is best used with the advice of a health practitioner.

FOS (fructo-oligosaccharide, inulin) is a complex sugar that helps digestion, enhances the immune system, and aids the growth of **probiotics** (good bacteria, such as **acidophilus**). It is also useful in maintaining proper blood sugar and cholesterol levels.

fo-ti (ho-shou-wu) is a cardiovascular strengthener, is rich in **bioflavonoids**, and is used traditionally to increase longevity and is a major tonic for the kidneys. It improves blood flow to the heart, and color and growth to the hair.

free-radicals are unstable, reactive molecules with an unpaired electron that can damage the DNA of cells. (22)

GABA (gamma-aminobutyric acid) is an amino acid derivative that functions as an inhibitory neurotransmitter of the central nervous system. It has anti-stress, anti-anxiety, calming and relaxing effects. It has been used clinically for depressed sex drive, prostate problems, and a tranquilizer substitute without any addictive qualities. It is one of the most important neurotransmitters in aiding the control of all convulsive disorders such as Parkinsonism, cerebral palsy and epilepsy. (211)

galantamine is an extract from daffodil and snowdrop that inhibits the action of acetylcholinesterase (AChE), an enzyme that destroys acetylcholine, a vital brain neurotransmitter.

gamma oryzanol is derived from rice bran oil. It increases the anabolic efficiency of food, basically increasing muscle mass with less food, possibly by stimulating the pituitary gland to release growth hormone. There is also some evidence that it helps increase energy levels, overall stamina, and aids in tissue repair from injuries. (183)

garcina cambogia see **Citrimax**

garlic reduces high blood pressure, bad cholesterol, and fights all forms of infections and disease in virtually any location in the body. It can be applied topically for athletes foot, or eaten to ease chronic bronchitis. It has antibiotic, anti-microbial, anti-viral, and antiseptic properties. It also detoxifies the blood and improves circulation. (191)

gelatin is a protein that comes from cartilage and the hooves of animals. It is used as an aid for growing nails and in the manufacture of vitamin capsules.

genistein see **soy supplements**

germanium is a trace mineral with a very special relationship to oxygen: it is able to reduce free-radical damage while increasing the body's oxygen supply. All diseased states, or tissue degeneration, can be traced back to a common origin: hypoxia, or lack of oxygen. Germanium can be toxic. However, an organic germanium **chelate** called Ge Oxy-132 has proven to be virtually non-toxic. Germanium increases oxygen in the cells and tissues. It induces the biosynthesis of interferons and interleukins in the immune system. It activates special cells in the **thymus**, which increase cancer-fighting macrophage activity. It has been used in the past with good results for people suffering from candida, viral infections, and cancer. Germanium increases energy, brain function, stamina and endurance, and improves heart muscle tone. The usual dose is 30 to 100mg of the non-toxic Ge-132 form. (192,203)

Gerovital H3 (GH3) has as its active component, procaine hydrochloride, which comes from combining two naturally occurring products within the human body: para-aminobenzoic acid (**PABA**), and diethylaminoethanol (DEAE, which is somewhat similar to **DMAE**). Procaine is a strong anaesthetic known as 'novocaine' in dental work. Dr. Ana Aslan of the National Geriatric Institute in

Bucharest, Romania, used it for pain relief in the arthritic joints of elderly patients. She soon noted the greatly improved physical and mental well-being of these patients. For almost two years 15,000 workers between 38 and 62 were monitored throughout Romania, with over 400 doctors and 154 clinics participating in the program. All the subjects were healthy, but aging. Sick days declined 40% in this group, prompting the Romanian government to heavily subsidize the distribution of GH3 throughout the population of their country.

ginger is a stimulant, and aids in the utilization of other herbs. Ginger inhibits inflammation, breaks down protein, stimulates liver function, and is a tonic for the heart. It is effective for nausea, breaking fevers, and for motion sickness. It is anti-microbial and an antioxidant, and is helpful for hot flashes, indigestion, bowel problems, morning sickness and wounds. It helps in the conversion of cholesterol into bile acids, and can thin the blood. Use with caution if one is taking anti-coagulants.

ginkgo (ginkgo biloba) improves the circulation to the brain, and is used to prevent strokes. It also stimulates oxygenation as an aid to memory and mental alertness. It is good for depression and tinnitis (ringing in the ears), eczema, leg cramps, the heart, and the kidneys. It should be used with caution by people on non-steroidal, anti-inflammatory drugs (NSAIDS) such as ibuprofen, or who have a bleeding problem.

ginseng is the called the 'miracle herb' because of its many uses. Primarily, it strengthens the body and brings its functions back into balance. It also equalizes blood pressure, decreases the effects of stress, increases circulation to the brain, reduces depression, and strengthens the reproductive system. There are two major categories of ginseng: Korean and Chinese that are more stimulating and heating, and American that is more calming and cooling. **Siberian ginseng** is in a category all its own. (183)

GLA (d-gamma linoleic acid) is an essential fatty acid most commonly found in **evening primrose oil, borage oil, black currant oil**, and Mother's milk. It supports the PGE1 (prostaglandin series one) function that affects hormonal balance. GLA is used for arthritis, eczema, alcoholism, weight loss, cardiovascular disease, inflammation, brain injuries, multiple sclerosis, mental dysfunction, PMS (pre-menstrual syndrome), menopausal hot flashes, and many other conditions. (226)

glucomannan is a dietary fiber from the konjac plant. It reduces hypoglycemia, high cholesterol, obesity and certain cancers.

glucosamine (glucosamine sulfate) is an amino sugar used to create cushioning fluids and tissues around joints. It repairs damaged arthritic joints, reduces pain, and builds synovial fluids. It is easily absorbed into the bloodstream, and is necessary in the formation of skin, eyes, bones, tendons, nails, ligaments, and parts of the heart. It is used for inflamed discs, sciatica, and many forms of arthritis. It is necessary in the production of mucous as a protective coating in the urinary, digestive, and respiratory tracts.

glutamic acid is important in the metabolism of sugars and fats. It helps with severe diabetic and hypoglycemic reactions. It increases the firing of neurons in the brain and spinal cord. Glutamic acid aids in the transportation of **potassium** across the blood/brain barrier. It is used for mental and nerve disorders such as behavioral problems in children, retardation, and muscular dystrophy.

glutamine (L-Glutamine) is a brain fuel that can readily cross the blood/brain barrier (BBB). It is also found in high amounts throughout the muscles. It is easily converted to **glutamic acid** in the brain, where it assists in the detoxification of ammonia. L-Glutamine aids in the building and maintaining of muscle, and is beneficial for weight loss and body-building programs. Stress, disease, inactivity, and injury cause the muscles to release L-Glutamine into the bloodstream; supplementation can prevent consequent muscle-wasting. L-Glutamine can improve memory, alertness and concentration. It is helpful against fatigue, impotence, glaucoma, senility, epilepsy, schizophrenia, and retardation, and it also decreases sugar and alcohol cravings. It is used in the treatment of peptic ulcers, auto-immune diseases, and arthritis. (184,197)

glutathione (L-Glutathione) is a very strong antioxidant and anti-aging nutrient. It protects the liver, red and white blood cells, and lung and brain tissue. It is needed for carbohydrate metabolism, glucose tolerance factors, and it inhibits the production of free-radicals. It aids **Vitamin E** in the prevention of cataracts, strokes and kidney failure. It detoxifies poisons, the effects of radiation, heavy metal pollutants, and free-radicals produced by alcohol, X-rays and cigarette smoke. It protects the body from drug overload, and the ill-effects of chemotherapy. It also aids the immune system, and helps white blood cells in eliminating disease bacteria. L-Glutathione reduces the effects of aging. Levels decline with age, and the need for supplementation increases. A deficiency first appears with tremors and lack of coordination. (193)

glutathione peroxidase is an antioxidant and anti-aging enzyme that controls lipid peroxides, hydroperoxides, and hydroxylradicals in the body. The amino acid, **NAC**, can act as its precursor. It is one of the most important protectors of cells in the body.

glycerin is a sweetener derived from vegetable sources that is added to herbal remedies. and is as sweet as sucrose. It contains **malic acid**, an aid to digestion and energy, and therapeutically unites with, and removes, toxins.

glycine (L-Glycine) is an amino acid used for prostate gland and central nervous system health, and in the treatment of bipolar depression. It aids in the prevention of epileptic seizures. When taken in large doses, L-Glycine releases growth hormone (**HGH**), and it can be converted to **creatine**, aiding in the construction of RNA and DNA, and in slowing muscle and nerve degeneration. L-

Glycine is important in regulating blood-sugar levels, and in the treatment of hypoglycemia. It also helps repair damaged tissue, such as the skin and joints. (211)

goldenrod (solidago spp.) is an anti-inflammatory and urinary antiseptic, and is also a diuretic, expectorant, and astringent. It is used to treat diarrhea and internal hemorrhage, and, as gargle, for laryngitis and pharyngitis.

goldenseal root is the most remarkable of healing herbs. It is very powerful, and should be used only when needed, and not for long periods of time. It has powerful antibiotic qualities that make it useful for all forms of infections, such as sore throat, infected tonsils, ulcers, colitis, and vaginitis. It is used topically for skin infections. It should not be taken during pregnancy. It regulates menses, decreases uterine bleeding, reduces blood pressure, and has been used successfully in China to treat brain tumors. (192)

gotu kola is an Ayurvedic herb that is very good for improving the memory, increasing energy, improving physical and mental endurance, and for strengthening the vascular system. It is used for varicose veins and for relieving depression. It stimulates the central nervous system, and aids in the elimination of excess body fluids.

grapefruit seed extract is a strong anti-fungal that fights candida and other yeast infections. It is an anti-parasitic, and is used to purify water when camping. It can be purchased as a liquid or in capsules.

grape seed extract (see **proanthocyanidins, OPC's**) is a type of **bioflavonoid**. It is water-soluble, non-toxic, highly bio-available, and greatly increases the effects of **Vitamin C**.

gravel root (eupatorium purpureum) is used for kidney and urinary infections and stones, and for prostatitis, pelvic inflammatory disease, painful menses, rheumatism, and gout.

green barley juice is derived from the leaves of young barley, and is rich in protein, enzymes, minerals, vitamins, and **SOD** (superoxide dismutase). It is beneficial for digestive problems, diabetes, cancer and infections.

green lipped mussel extract is an aid for rheumatoid arthritis. It promotes healing, reduces pain and stiffness of joints, and inhibits inflammatory enzymes. It is high in proteins, vitamins, trace minerals, **SOD** (superoxide dismutase) and polysaccharides. It also benefits the eyes, skin, bones and intestines.

green tea is a strong antioxidant with anti-carcinogenic properties. It also protects cells from the effects of radiation, and blocks the absorption of cholesterol. It aids in reducing mental fatigue, and is available without caffeine.

grindelia (grindelia spp.) is an expectorant and anti-spasmodic used for bronchitis, sinus congestion, and bladder infections. It is used topically for poison oak and ivy, and for insect bites.

GTF see **chromium**

guar gum is a tasteless, gel-forming fiber that curbs the appetite, slows down digestion, creates stability in blood sugar levels, reduces the risk of colon cancer, and lowers blood-serum cholesterol levels. It is important to drink extra water with it, and it is available in powder or capsules.

guarana is a plant from Brazil and Uruguay which is high in caffeine, and is a strong stimulant. (202)

guggul (gugulipid) is an Ayurvedic herb that is used to lower cholesterol levels and increase white blood-cell count. It possesses strong disinfecting properties. Other uses include treating the common cold, inflammation associated with arthritis, and various skin, dental, and ophthalmic infections.

gymnema sylvestre is an Ayurvedic herb used to control diabetes by increasing insulin production, and is also an aid in reducing cravings for sugar.

hawthorne berry is a tonic for the heart and improves circulation. It inhibits free-radical damage, and prevents collagen destruction and inflammation. It is used to treat high blood pressure, angina, palpitations, and arteriosclerosis. It increases the availability of **Vitamin C** to the cells. Hawthorne berry has no side effects, but if one is using heart medications they should confer with their doctor before using it.

hemp seed oil is from the rape seed plant, and is a rich source of essential fatty acids. It is an aid to the brain, eyes, hair, skin, nails, and heart. It has anti-cancer, anti-inflammatory and anti-depression properties. (226)

hesperidin is a **bioflavonoid** found in oranges and lemons. It reduces capillary fragility, along with heparin in the liver.

herbs are the leaves, roots, stems, flowers, bark, and mycelia of plants used for health purposes. (20,231)

HGH (human growth hormone) is an endocrine hormone that triggers the body to replace the cells that die on a daily basis. It is produced in the pituitary gland. Aging reduces levels of HGH, which in turn reduces replacement of cells. HGH is a necessary link to strength, increased muscle mass, energy, sexual potency, lower body fat, and enhanced brain function. Every organ and system in the body is dependent on HGH for proper growth, function and development. **Deer antler velvet** and transferrulic acid are aids in the formation of HGH. **Arginine**, **ornithine** and **lysine** promote the release of HGH at bedtime when taken on an empty stomach.

HMB (beta-hydroxy beta-methylbutyrate) is a metabolite of **leucine**, one of the branch-chain amino acids. It aids in building muscle and reducing body fat, but only in combination with vigorous exercise.

histidine is an amino acid that produces histamine, a precursor to good immune response. It is used for countering allergic reactions, colds, and respiratory problems. It is important in the production of red and white blood cells, **glutamic acid**, and the transport of **copper** to the joints. It aids in the removal of heavy metals, increase the libido, and reduces headaches.

homeopathy A field of medicine that treats disease by administering a minute dose of a substance using the foundation of 'like cures like,' thereby using the body's own defenses to build resistance or overcome a condition. It will produce the symptoms of that disease, thereby building the body's resistance to it. (157)

honey is the combination of bee enzymes and nectar from flowers. It is high in protein, and contains vitamins, minerals and enzymes. It is excellent for sunburn, burns and wounds. Honey should not be given to infants under the age of one year.

hops (humulus lupulus) is a sedative herb used for insomnia, anxiety, stress, and in the brewing of beer.

horny goat weed (yin yang huo) is used in Chinese medicine for impotence, involuntary ejaculation, heart problems, fatigue, hepatitis and polio. It acts hormonally, and appears to dilate blood vessels. The active ingredient is icarin bioflavonoid.

horse chestnut (aesculus hippocastanum) is an herb used to reduce varicose veins and improve circulation.

horsetail is high in **silicon** and **calcium**, and is used to strengthen bones, tendons, hair, nails and skin. It strengthens the heart and lungs, and is helpful for arthritis, osteoporosis, edema and the prostate gland. It can deplete **Vitamin B6**, so that nutrient should be supplemented.

ho-shou-wu see **fo-ti**

huperzine (hup A) is derived from a type of Chinese moss. It is especially useful for treating memory loss in the elderly.

hydrochloric acid (HCL) is gastric acid necessary for proper digestion. A deficiency can result in gas, bloating, constipation, diarrhea and belching. After the age of sixty there is a greater need for supplementation, which can help ease the effects of osteoporosis, diabetes, and arthritis.

hydrogen peroxide (H_2O_2) is a substance produced naturally in the body which aids blood cells in the delivery of oxygen to the cells. It is also a germicidal agent that kills pathogens by oxidation. It destroys viruses, bacteria, and parasites. It is an aid in proper cell division, an excellent antibiotic, and eliminator of toxins. It is balanced by taking it with **SOD** (superoxide dismutase) and **catalase**.

IGF (insulin-like growth factors) are multifunctional polypeptides that improve energy, physical performance, and respiration. They also relieve symptoms of PMS and menopause, joint stiffness, and inflammation. They improve mental concentration, clarity, and appetite. Insulin-like growth factor-1 (IGF1) is released by many different tissues throughout the body, and creates potent anabolic and cell-growth effects. Production of this substance decreases with age. It is primarily secreted by the liver in response to a signal from human growth hormone (**HGH**), and, in healthy individuals, it enhances physical and mental performance, and increases physical endurance. The best sources are **colostrum** and **deer antler velvet**.

inosine is an amino acid metabolite, that has a unique ability to increase cellular energy, and is closely related to ATP structurally. No oxygen is required for this conversion, and it is the quickest pathway for the cell to get an energy boost. It works best when taken on an empty stomach with an electrolyte mixture containing **Vitamin C** and **CoQ-10** before exercise. This enhances oxygen transport throughout the system, improves workload efficiency, and prevents an increase in uric acid production. (177,198)

inositol (inositol phosphate, inositol hexaphosphate) is necessary for normal growth and maturation, especially of the liver and bone marrow cells. It acts as an emulsifier, digesting and absorbing fats in the blood. It is necessary for the myelin sheath around nerves and helps brain function during drug withdrawal. It inhibits the growth of certain tumors, is helpful in nerve diseases caused by diabetes, is effective against panic attacks, and has anti-depressant effects. Inositol is necessary for the proper action of neurotransmitters such as serotonin and acetylcholine. Inositol has no RDA, but the recommended dose is 300mg daily. The therapeutic dose is 1000 to as high as 12,000mg for certain conditions. Frequently, one finds **choline** and inositol combined in a single supplement.

inositol hexanicotinate (IP6) is a form of niacin (**Vitamin B3**) and **inositol** that has shown to have certain anti-cancer and cholesterol-lowering properties.

iodine is needed for a healthy thyroid gland, which creates the thyroid hormones. Iodine deficiency results in goiter (a swelling of the thyroid gland in the neck) and cretinism (retardation of mental processes). Excess iodine can result in acne and swelling of the thyroid gland. Iodine is usually found in **kelp**. The RDA for iodine is 150mcg, 175mcg for pregnant women, and 200mcg for nursing mothers. Generally, the range of iodine is up to 500mcg, with therapeutic short-term dosages ranging from 1,500mcg, up to as high as 250mg under clinical supervision.

ipriflavone see **isoflavones**

irish moss is a sea vegetable high in trace minerals and vitamins. It is useful for bad breath, coughs, and digestion. It aids the kidneys and heart. and helps to dissolve fat. It is an emollient and demulcent.

iron is essential for life. It is necessary for the production of hemoglobin and the oxygenation of red blood cells. Iron deficiency is the most common nutrient deficiency in the United States, especially among infants, teenage girls, pregnant women and the elderly. Iron is important for immunity, growth, stress, and for general well-being. Iron-containing products should be kept well out of the reach of children; it is a leading cause of fatal poisoning in children under six. Iron, in the form of ferrous sulfate, is an inferior form because it causes constipation and reduces **Vitamin E** levels. Ferrous fumarate does not cause this problem, but can cause stomach upset. Ferrous triglycinate and bisglycinate are very gentle on the stomach, enhance **Vitamin E** absorption, and do not cause constipation. There is a peptonate form that is easily absorbed, as is the ferronyl carbonyl form. The RDA is 10mg for men, 18mg for women, and 30mg for pregnant women. In general, men need much less iron than women. Women require more iron because of blood loss during menstruation. Iron is stored in the liver, and excessive amounts can become very toxic.

isoflavones are phyto-estrogens commonly found in soybeans and other legumes. They strengthen bones, counter the effects of chemotherapy, and control excess estrogen. They are anti-inflammatory, anti-cancer, blocking angiogenesis (stopping blood to tumors), and aiding proper circulation. Some isoflavones are **genistein** and **daidzen**.

isoleucine (L-Isoleucine) is usually used in conjunction with **leucine** and **valine**, the two other branch-chained amino acids. These three are often used by athletes to increase endurance, rebuild damaged tissue, and to increase energy levels. L-

Isoleucine is essential for hemoglobin formation and the regulation of blood sugar. When taken, this amino acid needs to be balanced one part **leucine** to two parts **valine** and L-Isoleucine. (180)

ivy (hedera helix) is an evergreen vine that is an anti-spasmodic. It supports the health of the lungs and the bronchial passageways in the respiratory system.

jamaican dogwood (piscidia erythrina) is a sedative herb used for migraines, insomnia, and menstrual cramps.

kava kava induces mental relaxation and aids in the reduction of stress, anxiety and nervousness. It appears to be helpful with urinary tract infections and insomnia. It should not be used by those with Parkinsonism, or with alcohol, since it can cause drowsiness. Long term and excessive use can cause skin problems, and it has been linked to liver problems.

kelp contains high amounts of trace minerals and **iodine**. It dramatically reduces the amount of radiation absorbed by bone tissue. It acts as an antibiotic, reduces cholesterol, and aids in the prevention of breast cancer by enhancing the immune system.

kombucha tea (Manchurian mushroom) is composed of bacteria, lichen and yeast. One only drinks the liquid extract. It is an energizer, a detoxifier, and appears to be useful for cancer and multiple sclerosis.

kudzu is an herb that contains **daidzen** and daidzein which relieves, and can prevent, hangovers from alcohol. It is also an aid in the treatment of alcoholism. The dose is 1000-1500mg either before or after drinking alcohol.

lactase is an enzyme that converts lactose (milk sugar) into glucose and galactose. Supplementation of this enzyme aids those who are lactose-intolerant.

lactoferrin helps maintain the friendly flora (bacteria) in the intestines, while it attacks harmful bacteria. It is able to bind great amounts of excess **iron** in the body. It is derived from cow's milk.

larch tree contains natural arabinogalactans which act as food for friendly bacteria in the gut, and as a strong aid to the immune system.

lecithin is the dietary source of **phosphatidyl choline** and phosphatydyl ethanolamine. It is also a good source of **inositol**. It lowers serum cholesterol, acts as an emulsifier of fats, aids brain function, and is a major component of the mylein sheath and the brain. (193)

lemon balm (melissa) is an herb used for fevers, anxiety and depression. It aids digestion, and can be used topically for cold sores.

leucine (L-Leucine) is an amino acid that speeds tissue and bone healing, and is excellent for convalescence after surgery. It decreases elevated blood-sugar levels, and increases growth hormone production. However, excessive use can form ammonia in the body and worsen hypoglycemia. (180)

licorice is an herb used as a tonic for the heart and spleen, and for treating ulcers, colds, and skin problems. It is useful for the eyes, reducing the possibility of cataracts. It strengthens the immune system, purifies the liver and blood, and reduces hypoglycemia. It is helpful in many disease conditions, from rheumatoid arthritis and asthma, to loss of skin pigmentation. It is helpful in eczema, cancer, celiac disease, chronic fatigue syndrome, herpes, lyme disease, lupus, and measles. It is also an expectorant used for coughs and congestion. It has estrogen and **progesterone**-like properties. It stimulates interferon production, and regulates blood sugar. It should be avoided by people with high blood pressure.

lignin is a fiber that binds with and removes bile and cholesterol. It is beneficial for preventing gallstones, and is an aid against cancer and diabetes. It can be found in **flax seed** oil.

linoleic acid see **CLA**

lion's mane (hericium erinaceus) produces eninacines which stimulate neurons to re-grow, aiding muscular coordination, brain function, and nerve response.

lipase is an enzyme for the proper digestion of fats. It aids in the control of LDL (bad) cholesterol, and is helpful in lowering high levels of triglycerides in the blood. Lipase helps digest fat-soluble vitamins, and balances fatty acids. Lipase deficiencies create a tendency towards difficulty losing weight, skin problems, high cholesterol, high triglycerides, and diabetes.

lipotropics help emulsify fats, making them readily transportable in the blood. **Phosphatidyl choline** and **choline** increase the production of **lecithin** in the liver. **Methionine** and **inositol** help detoxify the waste-products of protein breakdown, which is very important for those on high protein diets. (184)

lithium is a trace mineral that works with sodium metabolism in the nerves and muscles of the body. It calms the nervous system, and has a helpful effect on the psychological state of the mind. It is also beneficial for the heart, digestion and kidneys. A deficiency can result in birth defects, attention deficit disorder (ADD), depression, suicide, paranoid schizophrenia, and many other psychological problems which are aggravated by high sugar usage.

liver is an organ meat that promotes strength, endurance and physical stamina. It contains large amounts of **B-Complex** vitamins, as well as many other nutrients. (184,193,201)

lobelia is an herb used as an emetic and cough suppressant. It is used historically for asthma, bronchitis, and whooping cough.

lomatium (lomatium dissectum) is an herb with anti-viral properties. It is used for Epstein-Barr virus, genital warts, and many other immune-deficiency problems.

lutein is a carotenoid pigment found in many green vegetables, and is usually derived from marigold flower petals. Researchers have found that adults who consume 6mg of lutein daily show a significant decrease in their risk of developing macular degeneration of the eyes. Even normal-sighted people who take lutein supplements report reduced glare and sharper vision. This can be helpful for anyone exposed to brilliant sunlight or computer screens on a daily basis. Lutein does not have the **Vitamin A** activity of **beta carotene,** and competes with it for absorption and transportation. Therefore, it is wise to take these two nutrients each day at different meals. Absorption is enhanced when taken with good oils that produce the HDL form of cholesterol. All carotenoids require a small amount of dietary fat for absorption.

lycopene is a red carotenoid from watermelon and tomatoes. It is especially beneficial for the prostate and testicles. It protects against breast, skin and prostate cancer. It is a very potent antioxidant, detoxifier, and helps inhibit the production of cholesterol.

lysine (L-Lysine) is an essential amino acid that is a vital building block of all proteins. It is necessary for proper growth and bone development, and reduces **calcium** loss in the urine. L-Lysine aids in the production of hormones, collagen and enzymes. It is essential to the nervous system, and is used to treat

Parkinsonism, hypothyroidism and Alzheimer's. It aids in the production of antibodies, and inhibits viral infections. It is recommended for herpes simplex, cankers and cold sores.

ma huang see **ephedra**

maca (Peruvian ginseng) is rich in sugars, protein, starches and essential minerals, including **iodine** and **iron**. It was traditionally used by the Aztecs to enhance fertility. Today, it is taken to promote energy, stamina, endurance, mental clarity, and to help balance female hormones.

magnesium is a component of every cell, and is vital to many enzyme systems. It activates most of the **B-Complex** vitamins, is involved in the production and transfer of energy for protein synthesis, and is required for proper nerve function and contraction of muscles. It also affects the action of various hormones and cellular electrolyte content. It is involved in over six hundred metabolic processes. The most basic form is magnesium oxide, which is easily absorbed, but can frequently be the cause of diarrhea for some individuals. Magnesium gluconate is better absorbed, but also can result in diarrhea if too much is taken. Other excellent **chelated** forms, in approximate order of assimilation from less to more, are citrate, glycinate, aspartate, and orotate. Magnesium chloride seems to be especially beneficial for enlarged prostate. Magnesium malate appears to reduce excessive aluminum from the system -- aluminum having been linked to Alzheimer's disease. Magnesium taurate seems to be very helpful for the nervous system, and for nerve disorders. Magnesium has a RDA of 300 to 350mg. (15,204)

maitake mushroom extract fights cancer and elevates the immune system. It is often taken in conjunction with other mushrooms such as **shitake** and **reishi**.

malic acid is an **alpha hydroxy acid** from fruits and vegetables. It reduces hypoxia (the breakdown of oxygen to muscles), aiding endurance and stamina. It is also useful in fibromyalgia where it has been known to significantly reduce fatigue and pain.

manganese is essential for fat, carbohydrate and protein metabolism, growth and reproduction, sex hormones, bone development, healthy nerves, the immune system, and blood sugar regulation. Manganese is important in connective tissue development, and in the production of **SOD** (superoxide dismutase), which protects cell membranes from the attack of free-radicals. Manganese forms are listed in their approximate order of assimilation from lowest to highest: sulfate, gluconate, **chelate**, aspartate, and orotate. The unofficial RDA is 2.5 to 5mg. The therapeutic dose can go as high as 20mg daily. (194)

marshmallow is a diuretic and expectorant herb used for ulcers, congestion, sinusitis, and inflammation.

MCT oil (medium-chain tryglycerides) is derived from coconut oil. MCT's are shorter chains than most dietary fats, and do not require bile to be absorbed, and can go directly to the liver. MCT supplies two and half times the energy as the same amount of carbohydrates, making it ideal for endurance athletics, and as a protein-sparing supplement. It is soluble in biological fluids, and is not converted to body fat, but is burned for energy. If one uses large doses initially, MCT can cause cramping and diarrhea due to candida die-off. MCT is not recommended for children. (177)

melatonin is a hormone found in the pineal gland which controls biological cycles and immune functions. It is synthesized from serotonin, which is derived from

tryptophan or **5HTP,** and from nerve impulses in the eye as it is stimulated by light. It is useful in preventing jet lag, and is helpful in slowing the aging process. It is useful for **calcium** metabolism, menopause, cancer, immune function, and sleep disorders. It is a very powerful antioxidant, and is safe in large doses up to 300mg per day. Most products are 1-5mg taken at bedtime. It should not be used by adolescents, pregnant or lactating women, people on cortisone, or people with kidney disease. If vivid or disturbing dreams are experienced, use should be discontinued. It should be refrigerated since it is very temperature-sensitive.

methionine (L-Methionine) is an essential amino acid that detoxifies the tissues and assists in **choline** production. It breaks down fats in the liver and arteries, reduces serum cholesterol, is a potent antioxidant, and regulates blood pressure. L-Methionine is an aid to the lymph system and the liver. It promotes the excretion of estrogen, and is necessary for the production of nucleic acids and **collagen**, therefore helping prevent hair loss, and keeping skin and nails healthy.

methionine reductase is a potent, antioxidant **enzyme** that requires the

presence of **copper** in order to
function in the body.

methoxy (5-methyl-7-methoxy-
isoflavone) is a bioflavonoid which
aids the body in the production of
lean muscle mass with no negative
effects. It improves the utilization of
oxygen, reduces body fat, and lowers
cholesterol. (185)

milk thistle (see **silymarin**) is used
in the liver to increase the flow of
liver bile. It stimulates the
production of new liver cells, and is
helpful for jaundice, hepatitis and
psoriasis. It is also beneficial for the
adrenal system, the immune system,
and for inflammatory bowel
problems. It has the ability to protect
the liver from mushroom poisoning.
It is found in the liver, bile, and
intestines, where it is a very
powerful detoxifier.

minerals are inorganic (do not
contain a carbon molecule)
substances essential for life. (12,194)

modified citrus pectin (MCP) is a
potent aid in fighting prostate, breast
and skin cancer, for which large
doses are required.

molybdenum is a micronutrient
which is involved in alcohol
detoxification, **sulfur** metabolism,
and uric acid formation. It is
relatively non-toxic, but an excess

can lead to **iron** deficiency. Molybdenum assists in moving **iron** out from the liver to be utilized by the body. It also blocks the action of testosterone and some other androgens, thus it may be helpful in hair loss and aging. Molybdenum appears to work with flouride in preventing tooth decay. It is beneficial against certain types of cancer, possibly due to molybdenum's role as a detoxifier of chemicals and other metals. Molybdenum is best assimilated from a **chelated** form. The suggested dosage is 200 to 500mcg. Amounts over 10mg may produce excessive uric acid.

monolaurin (lauric acid) is a fatty acid that inhibits viral replication without harming healthy cells. It is particularly useful for herpes, chronic fatigue syndrome, Epstein-Barr syndrome, and flu-like symptoms.

MSM (methyl-sulfonyl-methane) is a natural form of **sulfur** found in all living organisms. It helps form the bonds that link connective tissues together. MSM is used to relieve both food and pollen-type allergies, improve over-acidic conditions, and to control constipation. It can improve lung function, and help alleviate parasitic problems in the intestinal and urogenital tracts. It protects against lupus, rheumatoid arthritis, and breast and colon cancer. It reduces arthritic pain, relieves snoring, improves the growth and texture of nails and hair, and increases the elasticity of the skin.

muira-puama (nervine) is a root from a Brazilian shrub, used there as an aphrodisiac, and to treat both frigidity and impotence. Many people report that the energy from muira-puama is usually accompanied by a calm, centered, and almost steely quality of strength. (202)

mullein leaf (verbascum thapsus) is an expectorant and demulcent that reduces the effects of hay fever, and other allergic reactions.

NAC (N-Acetylcysteine) is an amino acid that is a precursor to **glutathione peroxidase** and is excellent in preventing the ill-effects of chemotherapy and radiation. It eliminates free-radicals, heavy metals, and other toxins. It helps create T-cells and other immune factors, and is an anti-viral which is especially beneficial in the treatment of HIV and AIDS. It protects bone marrow, lung tissue, the liver and kidneys. It is recommended in cases of cancer, rheumatoid arthritis, bronchitis, emphysema, and tuberculosis. It aids in the proper absorption of **iron**, and promotes the building of muscles, while burning fat. It promotes healing and hair growth. NAC does not require the addition of **Vitamin C** for stabilization, as does **cysteine**. Its immediate use can counteract damage caused by an overdose of the analgesic, acetominophen. (194)

NADH (nicotininamide adenine dinucleotide, co-enzyme 1) is derived from niacin (**Vitamin B3**) and is found in every cell. It is important for energy production, and is especially important for the brain and the nervous system. It reduces the symptoms of Parkinsonism and Alzheimer's disease, and promotes physical energy, concentration and memory.

NAG (n-acetyl glucosamine) is a source of **glucosamine** that is well-absorbed by people with digestive problems by acetylating various chemicals. It is beneficial in the production of cartilage in joints, and is used as an aid for inflammatory bowel syndrome.

neem (nimbin) is an Ayurvedic herb that has a multitude of uses, from insect repellent to the treatment of fevers. It is a natural moisturizer, anti-bacterial, and anti-inflammatory. It is used to prevent gum disease, acne and eczema.

nervine see **muira-puama**

nettle is very high in **silicon** and other minerals, and is a detoxifier. It is used for hair growth, anemia, hay fever and allergies, and for strengthening the reproductive and nervous systems. It is excellent for the skin and scalp, and for an enlarged prostate. It helps alleviate arthritis, stimulates elimination in the kidneys, and reduces excessive mucous in the lungs.

niacin see **Vitamin B3**

nimbin see **neem**

noni is an immune-system modulator, and has been studied for its possible anti-bacterial, anti-viral, and anti-cancer properties.

nopal cactus (prickly pear) is a digestive enzyme that aids the pancreas in the production of insulin, and strengthens the immune system. It is a detoxifier, controls cholesterol, and reduces weight by regulating the absorption of fats and sugars from the gastrointestinal tract.

nutritional yeast see **brewer's yeast**

oat bran is a fiber that lowers cholesterol, aids weight loss, and helps stabilize blood sugar levels. It also helps in the removal of plaque in the blood vessels.

oat seed (avena sativa) is an anti-spasmodic used to soothe and support the nervous system. It is also used for depression, insomnia, panic attacks, irritability, and anxiety. It is helpful in breaking addictions, and is often used as an aphrodisiac.

oat straw is used to treat anxiety, physical and nervous fatigue, and depression, and helps to promote healthy skin. It is also used for colds, especially if they are recurrent or persistent.

octacosanol has been identified as the component of **wheat germ oil** that improves strength, reaction time, and endurance. It is a solid white alcohol whose exact mechanism of action is still unknown, although some evidence suggests it works to improves the transmission of nerve impulses. (206)

OKG (L-Ornithine alpha ketoglutarate) is an amino acid compound which increases endurance, muscle mass, and reduces muscle recovery time, especially in heavy weight-lifting, and strenuous physical activity.

omega-3 fatty acids (see **fish oils**) are found in **flax oil**, **hemp seed oil**, salmon oil, and other fatty **fish oils**. They are unsaturated, and the most common are eicosapentaenoic acid

(EPA) which is used in the production of prostaglandins and docosahexaenoic acid (DHA) which plays an important role in brain and nerve function. (216)

olive leaf extract (olivir) inhibits viruses, bacteria and fungi. It contains oleuropein, an antioxidant compound, along with certain acids that inhibit the production of toxins from molds and bacteria. It also lowers blood pressure, inhibits heart arrhythmias, relaxes the smooth muscles of the arterial walls, and increases the blood flow of oxygen to the heart.

OPC's see **proanthocyanidins**

oregano is an herb in which the oil is a potent antiseptic against a wide range of fungi, yeast, parasites, and viruses. It contains **Vitamin C**, **Vitamin A**, niacin (**Vitamin B3**), minerals, and the phenols thymol and carvacrol. It is used to treat diarrhea, indigestion, coughs and bronchitis. It is also very effective against athlete's foot, psoriasis, and eczema. It is used for insect bites, toothaches and earaches.

Oregon grape root (mahonia spp.) is a liver and blood cleanser, and stimulates digestion and absorption. It is used for sluggish liver, hangovers, acne, and eczema.

ornithine (L-Ornithine) is an amino acid that promotes the release of growth hormone (**HGH**), and helps break down excess body fat. It also helps to build muscle tissue and increase endurance. L-Ornithine helps detoxify ammonia, helps the liver regenerate and metabolize fats, aids healing and tissue repair, and builds the immune system. It is important to consult a knowledgeable health professional before it is used by pregnant women, nursing mothers, and children, because of the potent release of growth hormone. Caution is also advised for use by someone with a history of schizophrenia. (179)

oryzanol see **gamma oryzanol**

orthosilicic acid is biologically-active inorganic **silicon**. It is the most bio-available form of **silicon**.

osha root (ligusticum porterii) is a strong anti-viral used for herpes, sore throat, colds, and flu. It is a bronchial expectorant, and has immune-system stimulating properties.

oxygen is required for life and proper body function. It is necessary for metabolism, and balanced body pH. Without sufficient oxygen, the body becomes very acidic and functions improperly. Oxygen levels are reduced when there is stress, lactic acid build-up, lack of exercise, and environmental problems. Oxygen products are available that aid in the reduction of harmful bacteria without harming beneficial bacteria.

oyster extract is a good source of the amino acid **taurine**, and of essential fatty acids, proteins, vitamins, and important minerals, especially **potassium**. It normalizes blood sugar, relieves angina, and helps the liver to metabolize fats.

PABA (para-aminobenzoic acid) has a specific role in **folic acid** synthesis. It absorbs ultraviolet light and is therefore helpful in combatting sunburn and skin cancer. Also, it is used to treat vitiligo (depigmentation of the skin) and, along with **folic acid** and pantothenic acid (**Vitamin B5**), can help restore hair color. PABA has no RDA, but the suggested daily dose is 10 to 100mg. Dosages above 500mg are considered possibly toxic.

PAK (pyridoxine alpha ketoglutarate) is a complex of **Vitamin B6** and **alpha ketoglutarate**. It enhances physical performance, normalizes blood sugar, and reduces lactic acid in the body. (177)

pancreatin is a substance from the pancreas that contains the proteolytic

enzymes, **amylase**, and **lipase**. It is
an aid in digesting protein and
carbohydrates. Pancreatic enzymes
should not be taken during
pregnancy, or when using blood
thinners.

pangamate or **pangamic acid** see
DMG

pantethine (see **Vitamin B5**) is a
derivative of **Vitamin B5**
(pantothenic acid) that aids lipid
metabolism by raising the levels of
Co-enzyme A, which is a co-factor
involved in the metabolic pathways
of carbohydrate and lipid
metabolism. Its function is to
increase energy production in the
cells.

pantothenic acid see **Vitamin B5**

papain is an enzyme derived from
the latex of papaya, and is used in
the digestion of protein.

para-aminobenzoic acid see
PABA

passion flower (passifora incarnata)
is a sedative, hypnotic, and anti-
spasmodic. It relieves nerve pain,
promotes restful sleep, and is used to
treat seizures and hysteria.

pau d'arco (lapacho, ipe roxo,
taheebo) is a very powerful anti-
fungal agent. It also acts as a blood

and lymphatic system cleanser, and is used to treat tumors and candida. It is a hard bark that needs to be boiled at least twenty minutes to release all of its ingredients. It is also helpful for those who suffer from AIDS, cancer, cardiovascular problems, and rheumatism. Fungi cannot grow in its presence.

peperine is an extract of black pepper that enhances absorption of nutrients, and improves metabolism.

peppermint (mentha piperita) is used for upset stomach, heartburn, nausea, colds, flu, congestion, nervous headache, and agitation. It also aids diarrhea and flatulence, and adds flavor to other herbal preparations.

peppermint oil is an herbal remedy used to treat irritable bowel syndrome.

pepsin is a proteolytic **enzyme**, and is the principle digestive component of the stomach's gastric juice. It aids in the digestion of protein.

phenylalanine (L-Phenylalanine) is an essential amino acid that is converted into **tyrosine** which is ultimately synthesized into dopamine and norepinephrine. These two neurotransmitters promote alertness, elevate mood, and help suppress the appetite. It is an anti-depressant, aids in learning and memory retention, and is a thyroid stimulant. L-Phenylalanine usually takes eight hours to metabolize, and is best taken on an empty stomach at bedtime along with **Vitamin B6**. Another form, D-Phenylalanine is a powerful painkiller, and does not incorporate into the body's proteins. It is especially good for chronic pain, such as from arthritis, migraine or menstruation. The D form is very expensive, and is most commonly found combined with the L form as DL-Phenylalanine in a one-to-one mixture. Pregnant women, people with high blood pressure, those suffering from phenylketonuria (PKU), pigmented melanoma skin cancer, anxiety attacks, or diabetes should not take either form. (198)

phosphatidyl choline (see **lecithin**) strengthens liver cells and helps an impaired liver to regain health. It is important in nerve and brain function.

phosphatidyl serine (PS) plays important roles in neurotransmitter systems, metabolism levels in the brain, maintaining nerve connections (synapses) in the brain, and various higher mental activities. Depletion of PS with age appears to be correlated with the decline of these functions. It can help maintain or improve cognitive functions, such as memory and learning, in mature adults. PS is especially indicated for people over fifty years of age, and for people who may have prematurely damaged brain cells due to disease, alcohol, drug use, pollution, or other causes. It is used as a lifetime supplementation for epilepsy, in support of conventional treatment. It also protects against stress hormone release. It is not recommended for use when pregnant or nursing without supervision by a knowledgeable health-care practitioner.

phosphorus is the second most abundant mineral in the body. It is necessary for bone growth, energy production, cell reproduction, and brain function. It is necessary for muscle endurance and performance.

phytosterols are plant sterols converted in the body by enzymes into human hormones.

picrorrhiza kurroa stimulates the immune system, and is an anti-inflammatory. It has been used in Ayurvedic medicine for hundreds of years. It supports immune function in general, and has a specific healing and protective effect on the liver. (194)

plantain (plantago spp.) is an astringent and expectorant. It is used to treat coughs, bronchitis, diarrhea, hemorrhoids, bleeding, cystitis, chronic catarrhal problems, external wounds, and sores, insect bites, laryngitis, and gastritis.

pleurisy root (asclepias tuberosa) is used to treat respiratory infections, bronchitis, pleurisy, pneumonia, and flu. It reduces inflammation, and encourages expectoration.

poke root (phytolaeca spp.) is an emetic and purgative. It cleanses the lymphatic system for tonsillitis, mumps, laryngitis, swollen glands, mastitis, and rheumatism. Large doses can be toxic.

polycosanol is a long-chained fatty alcohol that reduces LDL cholesterol, increases vitality, promotes physical strength and endurance, and improves muscle reflexes. It is an aid in improving sexual libido and performance, and contains **octacosanol**.

potassium acts to relax muscle contraction and is needed for a healthy nervous system and a regular heart rhythm. Potassium converts glucose to glycogen, and is necessary for protein synthesis. Most of the approximately 250 grams of potassium found in the body is in the cells, whereas most of the body's sodium is found outside the cell. Together they act to prevent cell destruction and shock, and to regulate fluid balance. Potassium chloride is well absorbed, with these other forms in their approximate order of assimilation: citrate, gluconate, aspartate, and orotate. Generally, the requirement for potassium in the diet is 2000 to 2500mg daily. Government regulations keep the levels at no more than 99mg per tablet for supplements.

potentilla (potentilla spp.) is used as an astringent, mouthwash and gargle for sore throats and gum inflammation. It is used to treat stomach ulcers, abrasions, sunburn, poison oak, fevers and diarrhea.

pregnenolone is the precursor to **DHEA**, **progesterone**, and other steroid hormones in the body. Levels of pregnenolone decline with age. Pregnenolone does not cause masculinizing effects in women because it is less likely to increase testosterone levels. Recent studies indicate that it may be the most potent brain nutrient ever found. It is excellent in preventing and curing stress-related maladies, a major contributing factor to chronic illness. The conversion of cholesterol to pregnenolone is aided by the presence of sufficient **Vitamin A**, **Vitamin E**, thyroid hormone, **copper**, and light, and can be blocked by too much estrogen, X-rays, ultraviolet light, unsaturated oils, and **iron**.

proanthocyanidins (OPC's) (see **Pycnogenol**) are strong antioxidants from grape seed and pine bark extracts. They protect capillaries, veins and arteries, and aid circulation, block cholesterol, and protect against blood clots. OPC's strengthen **collagen**, and help to maintain healthy skin, eyes, cartilage, bones, and gums. OPC's are also **chelating** agents for harmful chemicals and metals.

probiotics is a modern term for friendly intestinal flora, such as **acidophilus**, **bifidus**, and **bulgaricus**. (194)

progesterone is a hormone that plays a major role in regulating the menstrual cycle. It enhances mood, helps protect against certain cancers, and reduces or stops bone loss (osteoporosis). It is important to know the proper time and dosage which varies with different circumstances. (see **pregnenolone**)

proline (L-Proline) is an amino acid that strengthens joints and tendons, promotes repair of cartilage, and aids the production of **collagen**. It works in conjunction with **Vitamin C** and **lysine** to strengthen the heart, arteries and veins. It helps to promote smooth, youthful skin, and flexibility. (178)

propolis is an anti-bacterial, anti-viral, anti-fungal agent, and has antiseptic properties. Bees gather it from plants and use it to maintain a sterile environment in their hives. It is used for pain, and for all forms of infections, especially sore throat. It is helpful in treating herpes zoster. (195)

protease is an enzyme that meets the digestive and metabolic needs of the body. It dissolves almost all proteins which are not components of living cells, and breaks down undigested proteins, toxins and cellular debris. It dissolves the outer coating of viruses, and reduces stress on the immune system. It can be taken on an empty stomach to in crease its proteolytic action.

psyllium husk is a mucilaginous fiber that acts as a laxative and intestinal cleanser.

psyllium seed is a bulking agent, and is a very effective cleanser of the intestinal tract.

pumpkin seeds are a source of essential fatty acids, **zinc**, and **B-Complex** vitamins. They benefit the prostate gland and the reproductive system. (226)

Pycnogenol (see **proanthocyanidins**) is the trade name of a patented extract from

French pine bark that is a highly active **bioflavonoid**, and is a powerful free-radical scavenger, even stronger than well-established antioxidants such as **Vitamin C** and **Vitamin E**. It has anti-aging properties, and helps relieve inflammatory conditions such as arthritis and sports-related injuries. Pycnogenol also repairs damaged **collagen**, and protects it against further attack by free-radicals. It improves peripheral circulation and strengthens weak blood vessels, including fragile capillaries. Pycnogenol helps prevent bruising, and reduces varicose veins. (195)

pygeum africanum is an herb from an African evergreen that reduces the symptoms of benign prostate hypertrophy and can possibly act as an aphrodisiac.

pyridoxine see **Vitamin B6**

pyruvate is a by-product of metabolism that triggers the release of ATP (adenosine triphosphate), the fuel for energy within the cells. It burns fat, promotes muscle tone, lowers cholesterol, and reduces blood pressure.

quercitin is a **bioflavonoid** that blocks histamine release in allergic reactions, and strengthens capillaries. It has been labeled 'mutagenic' by the controversial Ames Test, whose validity is disputed. It is considered effective for inflammation. (195)

red clover flower (trifolium pratense) is a blood cleanser used for childhood eczema, psoriasis, coughs, bronchitis, ulcers, inflammation and infection. The extract is also used for menopause problems and prostate health.

red raspberry leaf (rhubus idaeus) also called the pregnancy herb, relieves nausea, eases painful menses, reduces hemorrhage, and is a uterine tonic. It is also a remedy for childhood diarrhea, and a gargle for sore throat and bleeding gums.

red root (cesnothus americanus) is a lymphatic remedy used for tonsillitis, sore throat, enlarged lymph nodes and spleen, and for fibrous cysts. It is a mild expectorant.

red wine polyphenols are antioxidants that reduce the buildup of plaque in the arteries through the oxidation of cholesterol. They also protect against certain cancers, and reduce the formation of blood clots.

red yeast rice is a food that promotes the proper balance of cholesterol and triglycerides. Most cholesterol is synthesized in the liver; it is controlled by the enzyme HMG-CoA (Hydroxymethyl-glutaryl CoA) reductase. This enzyme increases when the liver senses more cholesterol is needed. The HMG-CoA reductase inhibitors in red yeast emulate this natural process to help maintain normal cholesterol levels.

reishi mushroom (ganoderma lucidum) relieves stress and soothes the nervous system. It stimulates the immune system, and is an anti-carcinogen. It aids the heart, the circulatory system, the adrenal glands, and the liver.

reservatrol is an anti-fungal compound in grapes which stops the formation of blood clots, is helpful in preventing cholesterol from clogging arteries, and is an aid in reducing skin cancer and leukemia.

retinol see **Vitamin A**

rhodiola root (rhodiola rosea, gold root, arctic root) is a potent adaptogen used for extra energy, reducing fatigue, and increasing brain function. It improves peak performance of muscle strength, endurance, and mental concentration. It is useful for depression and stress, and aids the heart.

rhus tox is a homeopathic remedy derived from poison ivy that is recommended for poison oak and ivy, rashes, hives, arthritis, chicken pox and shingles. It is used for sports injuries such as sprains, stiffness, and back pain.

riboflavin see **Vitamin B2**

ribose is a carbohydrate found in all cells that increases energy. It aids in the recovery of muscles after exercise, and increases endurance.

RNA (ribonucleic acid) is a protein that carries genetically-coded information from DNA to protein-producing ribosomes. Nutritional yeast is a good source of RNA and DNA.

rooibos (red bush tea) is a South African tea high in trace minerals, **alpha-hydroxy acid** (known to promote healthy skin), and anti-mutagenic components which protect DNA from harmful mutations. The tea is used as an anti-spasmodic for digestive problems and colic. It is an adaptogen that also aids nervous tension, constipation, allergic symptoms, itching, skin irritations, and mild depression.

rose hips (rosa spp.) is a mild diuretic and laxative, and a mild astringent. It is a good source of **Vitamin C**. It is used to treat colds, flu, general debility, exhaustion and constipation.

rosemary (rosmarinus officinalis) is a circulatory and nerve stimulant used for tension headache associated with dyspepsia and depression. It is also an anti-bacterial and anti-fungal. It is used externally for muscular pain, neuralgia and sciatica.

royal jelly has potent rejuvenating properties. It has high levels of **Vitamin B5** (pantothenic acid), other **B-Complex** vitamins, and biopterin, a powerful brain nutrient. The queen bee is fed royal jelly, and it is this substance that changes a worker bee into a queen and greatly extends her life-span. It is beneficial for reducing stress, clearing the skin, and increasing virility. (201)

rutin is a **bioflavonoid** which is a strong antioxidant and anti-inflammatory. It is useful in the strengthening of blood vessels, and in the treatment of hemorrhoids.

saccharomyces boulardii is a friendly yeast that lives in the gut and produces lactic acid, which has antibiotic-like action.

sage (salvia officinalis) is used for inflammation of the throat and tonsils. It should not be used during pregnancy.

SAMe (s-adenosyl l-methionine) is a metabolite of the amino acid, **methionine**. It is important in the production of the hormone, **melatonin**. It protects the cells from cancer, protects nerves from lack of oxygen, and is an anti-depressant. It is used for reducing arthritic pain, is an effective anti-inflammatory, reduces depression, detoxifies the liver, and helps treat fibromyalgia.

sarsaparilla root (smilax ornata) is anti-rheumatic, a diuretic, and soothes mucous membranes. It is also a blood cleanser used to treat psoriasis. The extract improves physical performance and balances the body's hormones.

saw palmetto is used for toning and strengthening the male reproductive system, maintaining good prostate health, and improving the function of the respiratory system and mammary glands. It also enhances endurance and promotes female fertility. It acts as a diuretic and stimulates the appetite.

schizandra (schizandra chinensis) is an adaptogenic herb used for fatigue and increasing stamina.

sea cucumber is an excellent source of **glucosamine** and **chondroitin** sulfate. It also contains a potent anti-inflammatory that promotes the healing of injuries. It is used for arthritis, bursitis and other bone and joint problems.

selenium is an essential micronutrient that acts as an antioxidant, and is as much as a hundred times more potent than **Vitamin E**. It is essential for normal growth, fertility, vision, and the development of muscle. It is antagonistic to heavy metals such as lead, cadmium, aluminum and mercury. Selenium is important for any disease associated with excessive oxidative reactions, including cancer, heart disease and aging. In viral cancers, selenium appears to inhibit cancer genes. Selenium is readily absorbed when derived from nutritional yeast. General requirements can be as high as 600mcg daily. The RDA is 55mcg for women, and 70mcg for men. At 1000mcg and above, selenium becomes toxic to the system. (196)

serine (L-Serine) is an amino acid that metabolizes fats, promotes muscle mass, and helps build a strong immune function by aiding in the production of antibodies and immunoglobulins. It can be synthesized from **glycine**.

shark cartilage is obtained from sharks caught for food. It is rich in mucopolysaccharides which are beneficial for arthritis, hemorrhoids and skin allergies. Sharks have a powerful immune system, and its cartilage contains an antiangiogenesis substance that inhibits the growth of new blood vessels. This seems effective in treating cancer and arthritis. It should not be taken by small children, and pregnant or lactating women, by diabetics, or by someone with a recent heart attack or surgery, unless directed by a health professional.

shark liver oil is a good source of **Vitamins A and D**, **omega-3 fatty acids**, and alkylglycerols. Alkyglycerols are an anti-fungal, help produce white blood cells, and aid in the elimination of heavy metals, especially mercury. They increase antibodies and other immune-system co-factors. The oil is used for healing wounds, cervical cancer, and radiation poisoning.

shepherd's purse (capsella bursa-pastoris) helps stop passive uterine or gastrointestinal bleeding. It is a diuretic and breaks up urinary stones.

shilajit is an Ayurvedic herb which helps accelerate processes of protein and nucleic acid metabolism, and stimulates energy-providing reactions. It also promotes the movement of minerals, especially **calcium**, **phosphorous** and **magnesium**, into muscle tissue and bone.

shitake mushroom (lentinus edodes) is an anti-viral agent, and an anti-carcinogen. It increases the production of interferon, which can reduce tumors. It also reduces cholesterol levels in the body.

Siberian ginseng strengthens the immune system, improves mood, and increases endurance, resistance to stress, and mental alertness. Check with a health professional if you are taking heart medication. (176,202)

silicon (silica) is the most abundant mineral on earth, and is important in bone and connective tissue formation. It helps regenerate the skeleton, cartilage, tendons, ligaments, skin, hair, and nails. Silicon aids in bringing about bone re-calcification. It also counteracts the toxic effects of aluminum, which is important in the prevention of Alzheimer's disease. Silicon adds strength to arteries and the synapses of the brain, and is essential in the prevention of osteoporosis. There is no RDA for silicon, however, 20 to 45mg is recommended daily.

silymarin is the active component of **milk thistle**, and is used for liver and kidney ailments. It increases protein synthesis and the regeneration of liver cells. It also protects the liver from chemicals, fats, insecticides, and drugs that impair liver function.

skullcap (scutellaria laterifolia) is a sedative and anti-spasmodic used for nervous tension, epileptic seizures, PMS, and for withdrawal from substance abuse.

slippery elm bark reduces inflammation, and is used effectively to treat diarrhea, ulcers, constipation, vomiting and cholera. It seems to draw mucous up and out of the lungs, and can stop fits of coughing.

smilax see **sarsaparilla**

SOD see **superoxide dismutase**

soy supplements contains many nutritional factors. Genistein blocks estrogen-dependent cancers. **Methionine** inhibits breast cancer development. The soy **isoflavones** of genistein and daidzein lower cholesterol, stimulate bone formation, help eliminate harmful estrogens, and reduce 'hot flashes' in menopausal women. Soy protein builds muscle, and maintains proper nitrogen balance while dieting. (185)

sphingo myelin is the complex that makes up the mylein sheath of the nervous system in the spinal column. It has possible benefits for nerve disorders and multiple sclerosis.

spirulina is a single large-cell algae; it is naturally sterile, seventy percent protein, and high in minerals and vitamins. It is an excellent source of **Vitamin B12**, **beta carotene** and **chlorophyll**. It is easily digested, controls appetite because of its high levels of **phenylalanine,** and is an immune-system booster. It aids in the removal of heavy metals, and is used to treat allergies, liver disease, cancer, cataracts, eye disorders, ulcers and senility. It is high in **phosphorus,** and needs to be balanced with **calcium** supplementation. (185,200)

St. John's wort is used to treat depression, but is also excellent for infections, wounds, burns, bruises, sprains, nightmares, and bedwetting. It is an immune-system stimulant, an expectorant, and an anti-bacterial and anti-viral agent. It can cause sensitivity to sunlight, and should not be taken with MAO (monoamine oxidase) inhibitors.

stevia is a non-nutritive sweetener many times sweeter than sugar, and is used in many countries as a sugar substitute. Bacteria that cause tooth decay consume stevia, but starve due to stevia's non-caloric content.

stillingia root (stillingia sylvatica) is an expectorant for bronchitis, a blood cleanser, and is used to treat skin disorders. Small doses have a laxative and diuretic effect, and large doses are a cathartic and emetic.

stone root (cullinsonia canadensis) strengthens the structure and function of the veins, and is used to treat varicose veins, hemorrhoids, anal fissures, and rectal spasms. It is a strong diuretic, and helps prevent and dissolve urinary stones and gravel.

sulfur is a pale yellow mineral which is very important for the maintenance of healthy nerves, hair, fingernails, and skin. It increases bile function, and acts as a body purifier and cleanser. Sulfur appears most biologically available through a product called **MSM** (methyl sulfonyl methane).

suma boosts the immune system, reduces fatigue, and strengthens the liver. It appears to inhibit certain types of cancer. It reduces high blood pressure, improves anemia, and is useful for AIDS patients. It is also used for building lean muscle tissue, and contains hydro-ecdysterone. (203)

superoxide dismutase (SOD) is an enzyme and free-radical scavenger that controls and removes toxins from the body. It is found in all the cells, and promotes energy. It is an aid in treating rheumatoid arthritis, cancers, the effects of aging, muscular dystrophy, and radiation poisoning.

tannates have been found to have powerful anti-fungal properties, including against candida. They can form irreversible bonds with lipoproteins on the surface of fungi, destroying the ability of its cells to adhere to the intestinal lining, and eventually killing them.

taurine (L-Taurine) is an amino acid that is needed for the normal development and health of the central nervous system. It is synthesized from **cysteine**. Disturbances in L-Taurine metabolism are seen in problems such as epilepsy and heart disease. L-Taurine deficiency has been shown to cause eye and heart damage. A naturally-occurring, free-form amino acid which is not bound to food proteins, L-Taurine is found concentrated in the brain, and plays an important role in bile formation, and thus is important in fat metabolism and blood cholesterol control. Japanese scientists have found that L-Taurine lowers blood pressure and decreases blood cholesterol levels. Sensitivities to certain chemicals and an impaired immune response may result from low cellular levels of L-Taurine. Electrolyte mineral balance in the cells is regulated in part by L-Taurine. (196)

tea tree is an anti-fungal and anti-bacterial agent. It is an effective treatment for virtually any skin condition from acne to warts, and works equally well for athlete's foot and spider bites. It can be combined with oils such as **Vitamin E** for topical use.

theanine is an amino acid found in green tea that aids brain metabolism. It reduces glutamate toxicity, and reduces stress by acting on dopamine and serotonin neurotransmitters in the brain.

thiamine see **Vitamin B1**

threonine (L-Threonine) is an amino acid that helps to control epilepsy, and aids in the formation of **collagen**, elastin and tooth enamel. It supports the thymus gland, and is an immune-system stimulant. In conjunction with **glycine,** it elevates mood and improves neurological functions.

thuja (thuja occidentalis) is an expectorant herb used for coughs, warts, rheumatism and menstruation.

thymus gland is located behind the breast bone in the chest. It is where stem cells from bone marrow undergo division and mature into 'T' lymphocytes, which can distinguish between the self and the non-self. The T-cells then enter the lymphatic system where they become part of the immune surveillance system. It is available as an extract to aid the health and functioning of the thymus. (196)

tissue-cell salts see **cell salts**

TMG see **DMG**

tocotrienols are a special form of **Vitamin E,** that is much stronger in controlling free-radicals. They are an aid in lowering cholesterol, reducing blood clots, strengthening capillary walls, improving the skin and hair, and protecting against cancers of the lungs, cervix, breast, and colon.

trans-ferulic acid is derived from **gamma oryzanol** to promote muscle growth and tone. It aids the production of growth hormone in the pituitary, inhibits free-radicals, and aids the body in adapting to environmental change and stress.

tribulus terrestis has been found to increase seminal fluid volume, sperm count, sperm motility, and fertility. It is purported to build muscle and increase sexual performance in both men and women. It stimulates male sexual prowess through a non-hormonal pathway by supporting the body's own hormonal feedback system.

triphala is an Ayurvedic herb that is a combination of three fruits and is a highly effective, yet gentle laxative that rejuvenates the membrane lining of the digestive tract, and helps reduce inflammation, as well as supporting liver function.

trypsin is a proteolytic enzyme formed in the intestine or pancreas of an animal. It breaks down **arginine,** and is used to fortify the functions of the pancreas and the small intestine.

tryptophan (L-Tryptophan) is an amino acid that the FDA has permanently banned from sale in vitamin stores, but is available by prescription. In the body, L-Tryptophan converts to the neurotransmitter, serotonin, which regulates metabolism and mood. L-Tryptophan has been used successfully to treat insomnia, depression, PMS, migraine headaches, schizophrenia, compulsive overeating, and alcoholism. It can reverse the ill-effects of nicotine. A deficiency in L-Tryptophan has been linked to heart spasms. For supplementation of serotonin, **5HTP**, which is legal and available, is recommended.

turmeric (tumeric, **curcumin**) is a potent antioxidant with anti-inflammatory properties. It helps to reduce cholesterol and arthritic pain, and prevent blood clots. It is beneficial for the skin and eyes.

tyrosine (L-Tyrosine) is an amino acid that is a precursor on the dopamine, epinephrine, and norepinephrine pathway. L-Tyrosine is important for brain function and helps reduce depression, headaches, food cravings, and anxiety. It aids in the production of melanin (skin pigmentation), and of thyroid hormones. L-Tyrosine has been helpful for people suffering from narcolepsy and chronic fatigue syndrome, stomach stress, low blood pressure, low body temperature, and Parkinsonism. It is a natural mood elevator. However, it is dangerous to take L-Tyrosine with monoamine oxidase (MAO) inhibitors because of possible unexpected increases in blood pressure (see **phenylalanine**). L-Tyrosine metabolizes quickly, and should be taken in the morning, and not at bedtime, or it will interfere with sleep.

usnea lichen (usnea spp.) is a strong antibiotic, anti-viral, and anti-fungal. It is used to treat internal infections such as strep, staph, and trichomonas. It is also used for pneumonia, tuberculosis and lupus.

uva ursi (arcostaphylos uva-ursi) is a urinary antiseptic and anti-microbial for cystitis, urethritis, prostatitis, and nephritis. It is also used to treat kidney and bladder stones.

valine (L-Valine) is an amino acid that acts as a natural stimulant, and is involved in tissue regeneration and nitrogen balance. It is used to treat severe amino acid deficiencies caused by drug addictions. Also, it is beneficial for the liver, treating anorexia, and in reducing elevated blood sugar. Too much L-Valine may result in hallucinations and nervous reactions in the skin. It is very important that the correct balance of one part **leucine** to two parts L-Valine and **isoleucine** be observed. (180)

valerian is a powerful anti-bacterial agent. It is used for insomnia, anxiety, stress and tension. It is also used to treat pain from menstrual cramps, rheumatism and migraines. It is useful for high blood-pressure, ulcers and irritable bowel syndrome.

vanadium is essential for normal growth, and is a co-factor for several enzymes. It aids in the hardening of bones, cholesterol metabolism, and blood-sugar metabolism. It appears to improve insulin action, and is popular for this reason with body builders. The most common form sold is vanadyl sulfate. It is usually taken in doses of 50 to 100mcg daily. There are higher doses available of up to 500mcg.

vanadyl sulfate is the best and safest form of the trace mineral

vanadium, which is involved in cellular metabolism, growth and reproduction, and in the formation of bones and teeth. It may be able to reverse diabetes, and seems to mimic the action of insulin by stimulating glycogen production and the transport of amino acids into muscle tissue, thereby preventing the breakdown of muscle protein. Body-builders have reported impressive gains in muscle size from its use. Some research suggests that the trace mineral **chromium**, which also helps control blood sugar levels, is best taken at a different time from vanadium.

vinpocetine (vinca) is an extract of the periwinkle plant, and appears to be an effective memory enhancer. It increases micro-circulation in the brain, which helps to remove toxins and bring in nutrients.

vitamins are essential for life and growth, and necessary for maintaining proper bodily and reproductive health. (10)

Vitamin A (retinol) (see **beta carotene**) promotes growth and the synthesis of protein, helps develop strong bones and healthy skin, hair, teeth, gums, and eyes, counteracts night blindness, weak eyesight and strengthens the nerves and cells of the eyes. It promotes smooth skin and healthy secretions of the mucous membranes, helps protect the body from chronic diarrhea and respiratory infections, and aids in maintaining healthy thyroid and adrenal glands. Vitamin A is stored in the body. It requires fat, **zinc**, and other minerals and enzymes for absorption. In fact, a low fat diet can result in insufficient bile reaching the intestines, resulting in ninety percent of Vitamin A and **beta carotene** being lost in the feces. The optimum dosage is 10,000 to 25,000IU daily, preferably in small doses three times a day. The RDA is 5000IU. Vitamin A is protected when taken with **Vitamin E**, and its curative effects are doubled. Vitamin A needs sufficient **choline** in order to be stored by the body, and the need for it increases with age. Toxicity may occur at 100,000IU per day. (188)

Vitamin B1 (thiamine) effects energy, brain function and growth. Studies show Vitamin B1 improves mental functions in verbal and non-verbal IQ testing. It aids mental attitude, controls motion sickness, and wards off mosquitoes, fleas, and stinging insects. It enhances circulation, and is important in carbohydrate metabolism and blood formation. Vitamin B1 is essential in maintaining good muscle tone, nerves, and organ tissue. It is necessary for growth, lactation and fertility. It enhances immune response, and stabilizes the appetite and digestion. Vitamin B1 has a RDA of 1.5mg for men and 1.1mg for women. A daily dose of 50 to 100mg is recommended. Therapeutic dosages are from 3000 to 8000mg per day for special conditions such as Alzheimer's disease. No toxic effects have ever been reported in humans or animals.

Vitamin B2 (riboflavin) strengthens the eyes and helps prevent cataracts and corneal ulcers. It is necessary for growth, red blood cell formation, and antibody production. It facilitates cell respiration, the body's use of oxygen, and the production of cellular energy. Vitamin B2 is beneficial in the treatment of acne, chronic alcohol abuse, psoriasis, Sickle Cell Anemia, hypothyroidism, and migraine headaches. Vitamin B2 has an RDA of 1.7mg for men and 1.3mg for women. The recommended daily dose is from 10 to 100mg. Although Vitamin B2 is essentially non-toxic, it is difficult to absorb in the GI tract, with limitations of 20mg per dose. Therapeutic dosages of 400mg have been used for people suffering from migraines. Even a minor deficiency appears to result in a marked deterioration in personality.

Vitamin B3 (niacin, niacinamide, nicotinic acid) lowers cholesterol by preventing its buildup in the liver and arteries. Niacin moves fat from tissues for fat metabolism, burning it for energy. It promotes healthy skin, the health of the myelin sheath (the protective covering of the spinal nerves), and good digestion, where it is also vital for the production of hydrochloric (stomach) acid. It is an aid in protecting the pancreas, and is necessary for the health of all tissue cells. Niacin releases histamine that dilates the blood vessels, which produces heat, redness, and occasional itching of the face, chest, back and legs. This flushing aids circulation, is temporary, and usually passes after ten or fifteen minutes. Niacinamide, another form of this nutrient, however, has no flushing effects. Many people dislike the niacin flushing and take the naicinimide form. Niacin also dilates the capillaries of the brain and other tissues. It can help to relieve negative personality behavior such as schizophrenia, depression, delusions, and dementia. Niacin can also help relieve acne, migraines, vertigo, forgetfulness, high blood pressure and diarrhea. Niacin, in synergy with **chromium** improves blood sugar regulation by helping insulin function. However, high therapeutic doses of niacin, usually above 500mg per day, should be regulated by a health professional, especially if that person is a diabetic, has peptic ulcers, high uric acid (gout), or a compromised liver. Pellagra is the deficiency disease produced by too little niacin. The deficiency symptoms are dermatitis, diarrhea, and dementia. The RDA for adults is 13 to 20mg. The average dose is 50 to 300mg. The therapeutic dose is 500 to 2500mg. In special cases, the dose can be as high as 6000mg. However, some individuals may experience side effects at 500mg. Time-release niacin can cause liver damage, whereas quick-release niacin does not. The FDA considers niacin both a vitamin and a drug. It is a nutrient that one should monitor carefully if using it therapeutically, especially at high dosages.

Vitamin B5 (see **pantethine**) (pantothenic acid, d-calcium pantothenate, panthenol) is an anti-stress vitamin. It prevents aging, cell oxidation and damage. It is very important in the formation of immune-system antibodies, red blood cells, is a precursor to cortisone production by the adrenal gland, and is involved in the synthesis of all steroids. It helps in treating depression, and it converts fats, proteins and carbohydrates into energy. Vitamin B5 has been used successfully in treating allergies, rheumatoid arthritis, and in lowering cholesterol and triglyceride levels. It has possible benefits in the prevention of graying hair. Vitamin B5 has a RDA of 10mg for adults. The usual dose is 100 to 250mg per day. The therapeutic dose is 100 to 2000mg, especially for rheumatoid arthritis. (178)

Vitamin B6 (pyridoxine, pyridoxal, pyridoxamine) is involved in more bodily functions than any other single nutrient. It is required for brain function, the nervous system, red blood cell formation, sodium and **potassium** balance, for RNA and DNA synthesis, and in amino acid and protein metabolism for energy. Vitamin B6 is a primary immune-system stimulant, is necessary for brain chemistry, and is involved in the conversion of **tryptophan** to serotonin (an important neurotransmitter in the brain that induces sleep and relaxation). Vitamin B6 can increase concentration, and help with twitching, lethargy and headaches. It is used to help alleviate nausea, especially in pregnancy, air and seasickness, and radiation. It works as a natural diuretic, is beneficial for asthma and allergies by inhibiting the release of histamines, and supports nerve cell health in problems of carpal tunnel syndrome, epilepsy (along with **magnesium**), and for neuropsychiatric disorders. Vitamin B6 is especially useful in protecting against damage from stress, smoking and environmental pollutants. It helps protect against hair loss, tooth decay, acne, eczema, dermatitis, and skin lesions. Vitamin

145

B6 has a RDA of 1.7mg. The suggested dose is 30 to 100mg daily. The therapeutic dose can range from 200 to 500mg. This dosage is a very safe range, but extremely large doses can cause nerve damage. (179)

Vitamin B12 (cobalamin) is essential for the formation of DNA, the myelin sheath of the spinal cord, and reproductive and blood cells. It is also essential for the normal functioning of all cells, especially in bone marrow, the GI tract, and the nervous system. Vitamin B12 energizes a person and helps relieve depression and fatigue, and aids people with hangovers and poor concentration. It has shown significant benefits for sufferers of asthma, multiple sclerosis and AIDS. It increases specific antibody responses, strengthening the immune system. Vitamin B12 is closely linked to **folic acid,** and has remarkably beneficial effects on low sperm counts and tinnitus (ringing in the ears). It also plays an important role in the metabolism of proteins, fats, and carbohydrates. Vitamin B12 is often marketed as tablets, sublingual (under the tongue), a liquid spray for the mouth, or a gel that can be applied to the nostrils where capillaries readily absorb it into the bloodstream. It is stored in the liver, kidney and other tissues. The RDA for Vitamin B12 is 2mcg. The daily dose most often recommended is 100 to 500mcg. The therapeutic dose is 1000 to 7000mcg. An injection of Vitamin B12 routinely contains 5000mcg. Generally, there is no toxicity with Vitamin B12, but a continual usage of high amounts may cause an overproduction of red blood cells.

Vitamin B15 see **DMG**

Vitamin Bt see **carnitine**

Vitamin C (ascorbic acid) (see **C ester, ester C**) is essential to **collagen** and elastin production, the substances that hold the body together. Vitamin C detoxifies heavy metals, repairs tissue, promotes healing of wounds, and produces anti-stress hormones. It is required for healthy gums, growth, and adrenal gland function. It is a strong antioxidant, working especially on the fluids of the body. It can also help recycle **Vitamin E** in the body. Vitamin C can directly destroy certain types of bacteria and viruses. It also can increase white blood-cell activity, and plays an important role in the biochemistry of the immune system. It protects against cancer, heart disease, arthritis and allergies. It controls alcohol cravings, and is an important factor in treating male infertility, diabetes, constipation, **iron** insufficiency, drug withdrawal, and in suppressing the HIV virus. It strengthens the lens of the eye, and increases oxygen intake. Vitamin C is not stored in the body. We absorb the first 4000mg, and excrete any excess. The RDA for adults is 60mg. Most recommendations fall between 500 to 2500mg daily, with very reliable sources suggesting up to 10,000mg per day for certain conditions. One should add Vitamin C in slow increments when supplementing, and likewise reduce amounts slowly. Vitamin C is essentially non-toxic. Contrary to critics of Vitamin C, no cases of kidney stones, and only a handful of cases of increased oxalate excretion with high-dose Vitamin C supplementation have been reported. Reports of Vitamin C destroying **Vitamin B12** have also been proven incorrect. A form that is stored much longer in the organs of the body is the fat- soluble form, ascorbyl palmitate. The metabolite form is called **ester C**. (181,190)

Vitamin D is mainly synthesized in the skin from exposure to sunlight, and works like a hormone. It is targeted for the bones, actively transporting **calcium** and **phosphorus** into bone cells. The kidneys, lungs, gall bladder, skin, liver, breasts, and parathyroid gland need it. Most recent studies point towards Vitamin D's benefit in osteoporosis, diabetes, and leukemia. Vitamin D can be absorbed into the blood only in the presence of fat.

Those rarely exposed to sunlight should supplement this vitamin. The RDA is 400IU; the optimum dosage is 800 to 5000IU daily. However, levels above 2000IU may produce serious side effects for some individuals, and use at this level should be monitored by a health professional.

Vitamin E is found in every cell of the body, where it prevents free-radicals from damaging the cell walls. It also prevents cancer, cataracts, and cardiovascular disease. It improves circulation, aids in healing wounds and repairing tissue. It is useful in treating fibrosistic breasts and premenstrual syndrome. Vitamin E protects the structure and function of muscle tissues, the pituitary and adrenal glands, the capillaries, red blood cells and sex hormones. It can prevent sterility in males, and protects the lungs and blood cells from ozone damage. The RDA for Vitamin E is 15IU for men, and 12IU for women. The usual dose is 400IU daily, with a therapeutic dose up to 1600IU. Synthetic E (dl-alpha) has been shown to be as much as fifty percent less effective than the natural form (d-alpha). There is no upper limit of toxicity for Vitamin E. However, if one is on blood-thinning drugs, Vitamin E can make those drugs more effective. It is very important to have your doctor adjust the drug dosage accordingly. Also, it is recommended to avoid Vitamin E two weeks prior to surgery. Post-surgically, it is an aid in healing, and in the reduction of scar tissue. (191)

Vitamin K (phytonadione, phyllo-quinone) is essential for the normal clotting of blood. It is synthesized in the liver and intestinal tract by intestinal bacteria. It helps protect the liver in cases of jaundice and cirrhosis. It helps to stop bone loss, excessive menstruation, and promotes healing of broken blood vessels in the eye. It also acts as an anti-parasitic for intestinal worms. Vitamin K has a therapeutic dosage of 2mg. Most formulas contain much less to avoid any possible excessive clotting of blood.

vitex see **chaste berry**

wheat germ oil (see **octacosanol**) is high in many nutrients. It is important in the lowering of cholesterol, and improving the body's use of oxygen. It is also beneficial for Parkinsonism and muscular dystrophy.

wheat grass is highly concentrated vegetable juice; three pounds of wheat grass is comparable to seventy pounds of vegetables. It increases energy, and is a powerful detoxifier.

It is very high in antioxidant enzymes.

wheat sprouts are high in nutrients. Some specially-grown sprouts enhance the body's levels of **SOD** (superoxide dismutase), **catalase, methionine reductase** and **glutathione peroxidase** -- all very potent antioxidant enzymes. It is very beneficial for increasing energy, reducing free-radicals in synovial fluids around joints, and reducing the harmful effects of radiation poisoning.

whey protein is an excellent source of protein, immune factors, and antioxidants. It is derived from milk protein, but does not contain fat or lactose. It does have a number of growth and immune factors that make it highly effective for fighting infections. It raises blood levels of **glutathione** that protect against degenerative diseases. It aids in the rebuilding of the body after illness, and studies indicate it may extend life. (185)

white oak (quercus alba) is an astringent herb used historically in the treatment of hemorrhoids and diarrhea.

white willow bark is used for headaches, neuralgia, fevers, arthritis and rheumatism. It works like aspirin, and is the source for salicin, the pain reliever found in that drug. It has anti-inflammatory and astringent properties. Like aspirin, it thins the blood, and should be used with caution by those taking anti-coagulents.

wild cherry bark (prunus virg.) is an expectorant, anti-tussive, astringent, sedative, and digestive bitter. It is used for irritating coughs, bronchitis and asthma.

wild indigo root (aptisia tinctoria) is a lymph cleanser for local infections such as sore throat, laryngitis, tonsillitis, pharyngitis, mouth ulcers, gingivitis, and pyorrhea. It is best used in small amounts. Exercise caution, as large doses may be toxic.

wild lettuce (lactuca serriola) is a sedative, muscle relaxant, calms restlessness and anxiety, and subdues irritating coughs.

wild yam root (dioscorea villosa) is an anti-spasmodic and anti-inflammatory used for intestinal colic, diverticulitis, painful menses, arthritis, flatulence, and ovarian and uterine pain.

wormwood (artemisia absinthium) reduces fever, inhibits roundworm and pinworm infestation, and aids uterine circulation.

yarrow (achillias millefolium) reduces fever, lowers blood pressure, and is a treatment for thrombotic conditions associated with high blood pressure.

yeast see **brewer's yeast**

yellow dock root (rumex crispus) is a blood cleanser, and is used for anemia, hepatitis, and chronic skin disorders. It is a mild laxative, and aids fat digestion.

yerba mansa (anemopsis calif.) is soothing to mucus membranes, and is used for diarrhea, dysentery, malarial fevers, gonorrhea, catarrh, and digestive weakness.

yerba santa (eriodycton spp.) is an expectorant, bronchial dilator and mild decongestant used for chest colds, asthma, hay fever and bronchitis.

yohimbe is a very strong sexual stimulant that increases blood flow to erectile tissues, and is a hormone stimulant. It can cause severe side effects such as headache, dizziness and anxiety. Women should use it cautiously, and only in small amounts. It should not be used by persons with kidney disease. (203)

yucca is an anti-inflammatory agent, and is used to treat arthritis, osteoporosis, rheumatism and prostate inflammation. It is also a potent blood purifier, and is good for hair growth.

zeazanthin is a carotenoid from dark green leafy vegetables that is a potent antioxidant. It enhances vision, guards against macular degeneration of the eye, and retards the growth of tumors.

zinc is necessary for the health of the sex organs, and for reproduction, growth, and normal prostate function. It plays a vital role in the immune system, healing wounds, burns, acne, and easing rheumatoid arthritis. It inhibits viral activity, and allows for the acuity of taste and smell. Zinc needs to be balanced with **copper**, usually with 2mg. Zinc is a component of over eighty enzymes, more than any other trace mineral. Some forms of zinc are sulfate and citrate which tend to be harder to digest and can sometimes cause nausea. Zinc gluconate and picolinate are readily absorbed and easy on the stomach. Zinc aspartate, and orotate are other excellent forms of zinc that are beneficial for certain therapeutic uses. Zinc, more than any other mineral, can cause nausea if taken on an empty stomach. However, in the form of a zinc lozenge slowly melting in the mouth, zinc is well-tolerated without food, and is excellent for reducing the length of a cold. The RDA for

women is 12mg, and for men, 15mg.
The usual dose is 20mg daily. A
therapeutic dose can be up to 75mg.
(196)

<u>APPENDIX</u>

Homeopathy

Bach Flower Essences

Aroma Therapy and
Essential Oils

Sports Supplements

The Immune System

Energy Nutrients

Brain Nutrients

Stress Nutrients

Fats and Oils

Enzymes and Digestion

Herbal Glossary

The Regulation Controversy

HOMEOPATHIC MEDICINE

Homeopathy is a science based on restoring the body's vital energies. The remedies are gentle, safe, mild, non-toxic, and aim at stimulating the body to heal itself. They are among the safest preparations known to the field of medicine.

Homeopathic medicine is based on several principles:

The Law of Similars which calls for a minute amount of a remedy that creates a similar reaction to the disease or condition in order to increase the body's information to use in its defense.

The Minimum Dose Principle is the reduction of the active substance to the point that nothing remains except the vibratory information of the substance itself. The idea being that the less there is, the more the reduction, and therefore, more potent the remedial effect.

The Single Remedy Principle is the classical use of a single remedy at a time.

The Trigger Principle is when the remedy begins the healing process by stimulating the body's defenses.

The Antidote Principle is the use of the remedy in small amounts, and

157

increasing the frequency as the body first improves. Once the body is improving, the remedy is discontinued.

Homeopathic medicines are most effective when taken on their own within a ten minute 'before and after' block of time.

Homeopathic Remedies:

There are literally thousands of homeopathic remedies. The following are just a few popular ones and what they're used for...

apis Insect bites and stings, hives, runny nose, and joint pain

arnica Sprain, strains, falls, sports injuries, bruises, exhaustion

aconitum Cold, flu, children's earaches, fright

arsenicum Diarrhea, food poisoning, asthma, cold, runny nose

belladonna Sudden fever, swelling or sunstroke, teething, earache, menstrual problems, sinusitis

bryonia Bronchitis, chest colds, constipation, arthritis

calendula Cuts, lacerations, burns, abrasions, fever, sunburn

cantharis Burns, scalds, frequent or burning urination, sore throat

carbo vegetabillis Indigestion, gas, acid stomach, food poisoning

capsicum Digestive stimulant, joint pain, bruising, minor bleeding

chamomilla Teething, colic, irritability, earache, cough, runny nose, insomnia, excessive menstruation

cinchona Gas, indigestion, flu, sudden high fever, ringing in the ears (tinnitis)

coffea cruda Insomnia, migraine, neuralgia, restlessness, dysmenorrhea with pain spasms

euphrasia Hay fever, flu, colds, eye injuries, burning and watering of eyes

gelsemium Cold, flu, headache, stage fright, muscular weakness, dizziness

hamamelis Bruises, hemorrhoids, varicose veins, bronchial congestion

hypericum Nerve injuries, tingling, burning, numbness, asthmatic symptoms, excessive pain, insect bites, hemorrhoids, toothaches, depression

159

ignatia Grief, introversion, hopelessness, fearfulness, hacking cough, change of life

lachesis PMS, hot flashes, irritability, bloating

ledum Bruises, black eyes, rheumatism, gout pain, swollen joints

lycopodium Constipation, indigestion, to raise mood, psoriasis, gas, eczema

natrum muriaticum Colds, sneezing, water retention, weakness, fever blisters, dry cracked lips

nux vomica Irritability, nausea, vomiting, hangover, drug addiction, indigestion, bloating, heartburn, PMS, motion sickness

oscillococcinum A remedy for flu

passiflora Insomnia, nervousness

podophyllum Diarrhea, vomiting, gagging, headache

pulsatilla Colds, hay fever, childhood asthma, allergy, morning sickness

rhus tox Tendonitis, rheumatism, back pain, arthritis, sprains, hives, poison ivy, itchy rash, cold sores, colds

ruta graveolens Fractures, bruised bones, sprains, lameness, scalds, eye strain

sepia Herpes, PMS, eczema, hair loss

silicea Weakness, acne, poor assimilation of food, boils, constipation, weak memory, sinusitis, hay fever

spongia Wheezing, dry cough, asthma, hoarseness, laryngitis, exhaustion

sulfur Skin eruptions, colds, eczema, asthma-like symptoms, cramps in legs or feet

thuja Warts, moles, bedwetting, dry or split hair, scaly dandruff

urtica Insect bites and stings, burns, hives, eczema, vertigo, gout, sore throat, rheumatism

valerian Insomnia, soothes nerves, eases muscle tension

Homeopathic Potencies:

First, a mother tincture is prepared -- this is a potency of 1X. Next, the tincture is potenized by diluting it and succussing (shaking vigorously in a certain manner) the tincture.

Second, the potency is increased by 1X to 2X, (the X stands for a ten-fold increase). It is mixed with nine parts of alcohol and succused again.

Each time the number increases, the tincture is reduced by mixing it with nine parts of alcohol. At 6X, the liquid tincture has been reduced to sixty to one.

To create the 'C' potencies, the process is the same, but the dilution is ninety-nine to one instead of nine to one.

The higher the potency, the more powerful the remedy, and the less actual material present.

Low potencies are 6X, 12X, 6C and 12C. These are for body organs, symptoms, and acute conditions.

Medium potency is 30X, (30C is used much less frequently, and requires an experienced practitioner to prepare).

High potencies are 200X, 1M, 10M, and LM. These are prepared and administered only by skilled practitioners for deep action with very strict and limited frequency.

The Twelve Tissue Cell Salts:

The salt is followed by its source and then by the symptoms it relieves...

calcarea fluorica found in bones, teeth, connective tissue and skin.
Relieves: Rough, cracked skin, hemorrhoids, flatulence, varicose veins.

calcarea phosphorica found in bones, nerves, gastric juices.
Relieves: Bone problems, weak digestion, poor circulation.

calcarea sulphurica found in the liver, blood, bile, and skin cells.
Relieves: Skin eruptions, boils, and tender, bleeding gums.

ferrum phosphoricum found in red blood cells.
Relieves: Anemia, fever and inflammation.

kali muriaticum found in brain, blood, muscle and nerve cells.
Relieves: Head colds, croup, eczema and catarrh.

kali phosphoricum found in brain, blood, muscle and nerve cells.
Relieves: Mental fatigue, depression, insomnia, and nervous indigestion.

kali suphuricum found in muscle, nerve, blood and skin cells.

Relieves: Eczema, dandruff, itching, scaly skin and leg pain.

magnesia phosphorica found in muscle, nerve, blood, brain, and bone cells.
Relieves: Spasms and cramps, flatulence, headaches and shooting pains.

natrum muriaticum found in every cell and fluid of the body.
Relieves: Colds, loss of smell and taste, constipation and diarrhea.

natrum phosphoricum found in muscle, nerve, blood and brain cells.
Relieves: Excess acid, indigestion, and dizziness.

natrum suphuricum found in entercellular fluid.
Relieves: Water retention, edema, flu symptoms and acid indigestion.

silica found in blood, bile, skin, hair, bones and mucous membranes.
Relieves: Acne, boils, weak memory and excessive perspiration.

BACH FLOWER ESSENCES

Bach Flower Essences are preserved in alcohol, and are used to stimulate physical, mental and emotional responses. They are used for depression, anxiety, pain, shock, insecurity, and physical conditions such as eczema.

Here is a list of the negative quality to be dealt with, followed by the positive outcome:

Fright:

ROCK ROSE: Feelings of alarm, horror, and being intensely afraid. **Result**: The courage to face an emergency.

MIMULUS: Fright of specific known things, such as animals, heights, pain, and for shy, nervous people. **Result**: Bravery.

CHERRY PLUM: Feelings of losing control, of doing dreaded things. **Result**: calmness and sanity.

ASPEN: Vague, unknown apprehension and haunting premonitions. **Result**: Trusting the unknown.

RED CHESTNUT: Worry for others, anticipating misfortune, projecting worry. **Result**: Trusting to life.

Uncertainty:

CERATO: Distrust of self and intuition, being easily led and misguided. **Result**: Confidence to seek individuality.

SCLERANTHUS: Inability to resolve two choices, indecision, alternating. **Result**: Balance and determination.

GENTIAN: Discouragement, doubt and despondency. **Result**: Ability to take heart and have faith.

GORSE: Absence of hope, acceptance of difficulty, feeling pointless to try. **Result**: The sunshine of renewed hope.

HORNBEAM: Feeling weary and unable to cope. **Result**: Strength and support.

WILD OAT: Lack of direction or fulfillment, feeling of drifting in life. **Result**: Ability to become definite and purposeful.

Insufficient Interest in Present Circumstances:

CLEMATIS: Feeling dreamy, drowsy, absent-minded. **Result**: Ability to come down to earth.

HONEYSUCKLE: Living in memories. **Result**: Involvement in the present.

WILD ROSE: Lacking interest, resigned, having no love or point in life. **Result**: Arousal of the spirit of joy and adventure.

OLIVE: Exhaustion, loss of strength, need for physical and mental renewal. **Result**: Feeling rested and supported.

WHITE CHESTNUT: Suffering unresolved, circling thoughts. **Result**: Resolution to a calm, clear mind.

MUSTARD: Feeling that gloom suddenly crowds in, for no apparent reason. **Result**: Clarity.

CHESTNUT BUD: Failure to learn from life, make repeated mistakes, lack observation. **Result**: Ability to learn from experience.

Loneliness:

WATER VIOLET: Withdrawal, aloofness, self-containment, quiet grief. **Result**: Peace and calm, wisdom in service.

IMPATIENS: Irritation with constraints, tension, impatience. **Result**: Gentleness and forgiveness.

HEATHER: Longing for company, talkativeness, over-concern with self.

Result: Tranquility and kinship with all life.

Over-Sensitivity to Ideas and Influences:

AGRIMONY: Worry hidden behind a carefree mask, apparent joviality to hide suffering. **Result**: Feelings of steadfast peace.

CENTAURY: Being kind, gentle, quiet and anxious to serve, but weak and dominated. **Result**: Ability to be active and positive.

WALNUT: For protection from outside influences, changes and developments. **Result**: The link breaker.

HOLLY: Jealousy, envy, anger, suspicion and the urge for revenge. **Result**: Certainty that the conquest of all will be through love.

Despondency and Despair:

LARCH: Expectation of failure, lack or confidence or the will to succeed. **Result**: Self-confidence, willingness to try anything.

PINE: Self-reproach, self-criticism, assumption of blame, readiness to apologize. **Result**: Relief of the sense of guilt.

ELM: Faltering in responsibilities. **Result**: The strength to perform duty.

SWEET CHESTNUT: Unendurable desolation. **Result**: A light in the darkness.

STAR OF BETHLEHEM: Need for consolation after a fright or sudden alarm. **Result**: Comfort in grief.

WILLOW: Dissatisfaction, bitterness, resentment and feeling that life is unfair. **Result**: Acceptance without complaint.

OAK: Patient, persevering strength, and never giving in. **Result**: Ability to admit one's limitations.

CRAB APPLE: Self-disgust, feeling of uncleanliness, getting small things out of proportion. **Result**: The cleansing remedy

Over-Concern for the Welfare of Others:

CHICORY: Demand for attention, self-pity, possessiveness, self-love, feeling hurt and tearful. **Result**: Development of love and care that gives freely to others.

VERVAIN: Willfulness, stress, over-enthusiasm, fervor and insistence. **Result**: Quiet and tranquility.

VINE: Tyrannical behavior, bullying, demand for obedience, domination. **Result**: Ability to become a loving leader and teacher, setting all at liberty.

BEECH: Intolerance, fussiness, hyper-criticism. **Result**: Ability to see more good in the world.

ROCKWATER: Self-denial, rigidity, puritanism. **Result**: Development of a broad outlook and understanding.

AROMATHERAPY AND ESSENTIAL OILS

Caution: Even though many of these oils have great health benefits, some essential oils can trigger epileptic seizures, asthma attacks, or severe allergic reactions. They can reduce the effects of homeopathic remedies if used simultaneously. If one has a diagnosed health problem, they should consult their health-care provider before using them.

basil: stimulating and uplifting

bergamot: relaxing, uplifting, calming, antiseptic

cedar: meditative, calming, aids breathing

chamomile: sedative, anti-inflammatory, stimulates memory soothing

clary sage: for menopause, concentration, is euphoric

clove bud: antiseptic, energizing, soothes irritability, mentally stimulating

cypress: revitalizes, helps sore muscles, removes cellulite, is a stimulant

eucalyptus: decongestant, loosens mucous, increases circulation, stops infections, treats asthma, bronchitis and arthritis

fennel: detoxifying, tones muscles, suppresses appetite

frankincense: warming, centering, calming, healthy for the skin

geranium: system-balancing, stimulates the psyche, is a cell rejuvenator and anti-depressant

grapefruit: refreshing, purifying, rejuvenates hair and skin

jasmine: soothing and uplifting, relieves muscle spasms, has erogenous effects

juniper: effective for cellulite and muscle spasms

lavender: induces sleep, is calming, relaxing, healing, reduces depression, stress, and nervousness, cools burns

lemon: purifying, antiseptic, softens the skin

lemongrass: stimulates the thyroid gland, soothes headaches and tension

lime: purifying, stimulating and refreshing

marjoram: warming, calming, analgesic for pain and headaches

myrrh: meditative, strengthening, cooling

neroli: an aphrodisiac, purifying, calming, good for the skin

orange: refreshing,purifying, good for the skin

patchouli: warming, a nerve sedative, an aphrodisiac, an antidepressant, curbs the appetite

peppermint: stimulating, reduces fevers, decongests sinuses, soothes headaches and motion sickness, energizes

petigrain: aids the memory, stimulates the mind

pine: disinfectant, antiseptic, aids circulation, clears congestion, relieves anxiety, soothes mental stress

rose: is soothing, helps the skin, and reduces depression.

rosemary: stimulating, enhances memory and intuition, reduces joint and muscle pain, increases blood pressure

sage: for exhaustion, mental strain, cleansing and detoxification

sandalwood: soothing, meditative, good for the skin

spearmint: energizing, mentally stimulating, purifying

tangerine: calms and soothes, eases nervous tension

tea tree: anti-fungal, stops infections, promotes healing, an insect repellent

vanilla: soothing, calming, has aphrodisiac effects

vetiver: reduces anxiety, is calming, a natural deodorant

ylang ylang: an aphrodisiac, relaxing, improves creativity

SPORTS SUPPLEMENTS

Physical exercise takes many forms.
It can be strenuous or relaxing. It
can be aimed at cardio-vascular
benefits, toning, building, or training
the body for certain skills. Athletic
achievement is a worthwhile
personal goal, and good health habits
can produce positive benefits. The
longer they are practiced, the more
benefits one receives.

Some sports make heavy demands
on the individual which often result
in injuries. These sports in particular
require higher supplementation and
special products that help strengthen
the body in ways which can prevent
injuries and that can maintain intense
long-term activity.

What follows are several categories
aimed at the varied goals you might
want to attain in your sport activities:

Endurance:

Dimethylglycine (DMG), in the past
referred to as Vitamin B15, calcium
pangamate, or pangamic acid, is used
by Olympic athletes and marathon
runners throughout the world. It is
an intermediary metabolite useful in
the production of neurotransmitters,
hormones, DNA, choline, and
methionine. It enhances oxygen
utilization, reduces lactic acid
formation, and aids detoxification,

improving liver, pancreas, and adrenal function. DMG is especially useful for those who train to exhaustion or 'hitting the wall'. It delays the buildup of lactic acid in the muscles, and enables longer and more intense activity.

Siberian Ginseng, (eleutherococcus senticosus) is an adaptogen, a restorative of normal physiological function, allowing the body as a whole to respond to non-specific stress such as over-exercise. Siberian ginseng greatly enhances the immune system while simultaneously enhancing physical and mental stamina and endurance; it takes a few days for this substance to build up in the body.

Octacosanol improves strength, reaction time, and endurance. It is a long-chain alcohol which appears to improve the efficiency of transmission of nerve impulses. Studies have shown many benefits for weightlifters, swimmers, wrestlers, and track and field athletes.

It takes up to three weeks before the effects of octacosanol are felt. Once in place, there is an increase in the desire to exercise, as well as an increasing sense of well-being and strength.

PAK is valuable for those involved in both aerobic and anaerobic activity. It increases cellular energy as well as reducing lactic acid production.

Bee Pollen has a nourishing and energizing effect on the body. It contains the richest assortment of nutrients and amino acids of any substance known. Bodybuilders take it before a session to energize, intensify, and lengthen their workouts. It can be used at any time for quick energy, and is a substitute for coffee and other stimulants, while simultaneously nourishing the body.

MCT Oil stands for Medium Chain Tryglycerides, which are derived from coconut oil. They are shorter chemical chains than most dietary fats, and do not require bile to be absorbed. Therefore, MCT's can go directly to the liver. They supply 2.5 times the energy of the same amount of carbohydrates. MCT's are ideal for endurance activities, and act as a protein-sparing supplement. Since they are soluble in biological fluids, they are not converted to body fat, but are burned for energy.

Inosine is a nutrient that increases ATP (adenosine triphosphate) production within the mitochondria of the cells. It is so close to ATP structurally that no oxygen is required for its conversion. It is the quickest pathway for the cell to get its ATP. It works best when taken on an empty stomach with an electrolyte mixture, and with CoQ-10 before exercise. This enhances oxygen transport throughout the body, improving workload efficiency, and preventing any increase in uric acid synthesis.

Flexibility:

Proline is an amino acid which is necessary to rebuild soft tissue such as cartilage. It is enhanced in the presence of lysine and Vitamin C. Together, they greatly aid the flexibility of soft tissues, tendons, ligaments and cartilage.

Pantothenic Acid (Vitamin B5) aids flexiblity due to its involvement with the adrenals in the production of natural cortisone.

One of the most important factors in flexibility is being hydrated. Drinking water is the major goal -- not just fluids, but water. One of the finest waters to drink is 'catalytic altered water'. One good brand is Willard's Water, a product which can assure the efficient absorption of water.

Healthy soft tissue is kept toned by manganese and magnesium. Glucosamine sulfate and chondroitin

sulfate are excellent for healthy
joints.

**Building Lean Muscle and
Burning Fat:**

AKG, or alpha-ketoglutarate, is the
ammonia-free skeleton of glutamine,
and as such, can preserve muscle
during and after exercise without the
downside of loading the body with
toxic ammonia which can happen
when large amounts of glutamine are
taken. The best way to obtain this is
in the form of ornithine alpha-
ketoglutarate, which besides
functioning as an ammonia
scavenger and a ready source for
anti-catabolic glutamine, also
releases growth hormone, stimulates
insulin secretion, and ends up
increasing the arginine pool, another
growth hormone-releasing agent.

Arginine and **Ornithine**. Studies
have shown that these amino acids
can increase the secretion of growth
hormone, and many bodybuilders
report that they enhance muscle –
pump effect. It is recommended to
take lysine along with arginine to
prevent the outbreak of latent herpes,
to further promote growth-hormone
release, and to otherwise balance
other amino acids.

Vitamin B6 helps in the utilization
of protein foods, fats and

carbohydrates. It is best taken as part of a balanced B-Complex.

Leucine, **Isoleucine**, and **Valine**, branch-chain amino acids, have been shown to be the primary components of muscle protein. Ingesting increased amounts of these important nutrients during and after working out offers the muscle cells their preferred nutrition, helping exercise to increase muscle size and strength. This effect occurs in part because these amino acids provide a substrate for glutamine, an essential nutrient both for the muscle cells and for cell replication in the immune system, and in part because the branch-chain aminos are burned for fuel, sparing other proteins for tissue growth.

Carnitine is known for its ability to increase the utilization of stored body-fat, helping people to slim down and increase lean muscle mass. It is also considered protective of heart function, both because the heart uses lipids as the source of most of its energy, and because it helps to reduce blood levels of fat and triglycerides. Bodybuilders find carnitine especially useful when 'cutting-up', because it helps transport cellular fat, speeding the fat-burning process.

Chromium Picolinate has been shown to 'bulk-up' lean muscle-mass and cut down body-fat percentages.

There is also evidence that this supplement can reduce cholesterol levels in the blood. Chromium picolinate, as well as another form, GTF chromium, potentiate the action of insulin.

Creatine Monohydrate is a naturally-occurring compound produced mainly in the liver, and also involving the pancreas and kidneys. In human clinical studies it has proven to increase force production and muscle mass. It has been recommended for reversing the symptoms of age-related deterioration of muscles. Creatine supplements convert into phosphocreatine within the muscle, which is critical to the continued production of energy by donating a phosphate group to ADP to make ATP. Creatine can do this without needing carbohydrates, fats, or oxygen to recharge the ATP, which makes this supplement a source of powerful energy because it does not need to undergo a complicated process in order to produce it. It can also lead to the absorption of hydrogen ions released into muscles from lactic acid, which cuts back the 'burn' and reducing exercise fatigue.

Vitamin C is highly regarded by many bodybuilders. It is often forgotten that working out intensely creates heavy stress on the body, especially the immune system.

Vitamin C supports immune response and helps speed recovery from workouts. It prevents bruising, and promotes the release of subcutaneous water.

1-AD (1-androstene-3 beta, 17 beta diol) is a hormone that converts to 1 testosterone, which is seven times as anabolic as testosterone. It does not transform into an estrogen, thereby reducing water retention and secondary sexual feminine characteristics in men.

7-keto DHEA is a metabolite of DHEA which is more potent and is not converted by the body into androgens (testosterone) and estrogens. It has thermogenic (heat-producing) properties that aid in the reduction of fat while strengthening the immune system and enhancing memory.

Dibencozide is the co-enzyme form of Vitamin B12. Although already-buffed bodybuilders don't often notice much effect from it, there are numerous reports from ectomorphs (thin people) of a sudden and significant increase in energy, and the ability to effectively work out. This may be due to the correction of a long-term and marginal Vitamin B12 deficiency, which your doctor can determine with a simple blood test.

Digestive Enzymes may not be needed by 'genetically-gifted' bodybuilders, but for most of us, any help we can get in breaking down and absorbing our food is greatly beneficial. Without this process, whatever we eat is often wasted, which doesn't help build mass and strength. These 'bulking-up' enzymes can not only improve bodybuilding progress, but can also help to rescue one's social life.

Ecdysterone is a plant extract that increases nitrogen retention and protein synthesis. It is anabolic, and requires the addition of extra protein in the diet to be most effective. The usual dose for bodybuilders is from 80mg to 600mg per day, on a six-week cycle.

Gamma Oryzanol is derived from rice bran oil and increases the anabolic efficiency of food. It also increases body mass with less food, possibly by stimulating the pituitary to release growth hormones. There is also some evidence that it helps increase energy levels and overall stamina, and that it aids in tissue repair.

Ginseng. Asian (Panax) ginseng is the herb of ancient Chinese lore and folk medicine. The Latin name Panax derives from the Greek word panakos meaning 'cure-all' or panacea, a testimony to the wondrous reputation that has followed this herb for three hundred years. Most Panax ginseng is commercially cultivated in China and Korea in both red and white forms.

Practitioners of Traditional Chinese Medicine (TCM) consider Asian ginseng to be an energy tonic which is stimulating and heat-producing, and which increases yang energies. It is employed in a number of degenerative and 'wasting' diseases where chi, or vital energy, is deficient. It is contraindicated in conditions such as colds and flu.

The red variety is considered by traditional herbalists to be more potent and stimulating than white. Some scientific tests appear to confirm this notion. Studies confirm the stress-reducing properties, heightened endurance levels, cardiovascular, and other activities of Asian ginseng.

Glutamine is a primary nutrient for muscle growth, comprising over half of the free amino acids in muscle tissue. Studies have shown that muscle protein synthesis is highly correlated with the blood level of glutamine.

Lipotropics include methionine, choline, inositol, Vitamin B6, and betaine. These have been used by bodybuilders to decrease subcutaneous fat, perhaps by a process of emulsification. They can also help in the proper digestion and utilization of dietary oils.

Liver has been used by bodybuilders down through history for increasing stamina, muscle heat, and strength.

Methoxy (5-methyl-7-methoxy-isoflavone) is a bioflavonoid which aids the body in the production of lean muscle mass with no negative effects. It improves the utilization of oxygen, reduces body fat, and lowers cholesterol.

Whey Protein is an excellent protein for all uses, including strenuous exercise, bodybuilding, chronic illness, and convalescence. In the past, the prevalence of lactose intolerance has made it impossible for many people to use whey. Now, these products are available lactose-free.

High levels of quality proteins exert an 'anticatabolic' effect, meaning that muscle breakdown is prevented.

It contains large amounts of branch-chain amino acids (BCAA's), and the immune-enhancing effects of lactalbumin. Research has identified the branched-chain amino acids as the keys to both bodybuilding and exercise performance. BCAA's (notably leucine) are known to be directly oxidized in muscles, thereby acting as a source of energy. In addition, leucine is used for alanine synthesis in muscle; alanine is subsequently transported to the liver and used to make glucose, which is then available as a fuel for muscular contraction.

Recent studies have shown that lactalbumin, the main protein in whey, can enhance immunity in animals. Since strenuous exercise has recently been linked to the depression of immune responses in humans, it may be wise for athletes and bodybuilders to use whey as a major source of dietary protein.

Milk and Egg Protein Powders are excellent, high-quality protein. They are great sources of complete protein for those who can digest them.

Soy Protein is beneficial as an adjunct to whey protein. It is best used in rotation with other proteins, and at times in conjunction with digestive enzymes.

Spirulina contains around 65% easily-digested protein. This is a complete protein which includes all the essential amino acids and is high in phenylalanine. It has also been found useful as an aid to appetite suppression and 'cutting-up.'

THE IMMUNE SYSTEM

The immune system is a network of complex interactions at many different levels, involving the white blood cells, bone marrow, lymph tissues and vessels, the nervous system, and many different chemical components.

Since the fundamental tasks of the immune system are founded on its ability to distinguish between 'self' and 'not-self', it's not surprising that, in that case, the mind is so important. In addition to our state of mind, the fields of genetics, biochemistry, anatomy, pharmacology, pathology, allergies, infectious disease, organ transplantation, rheumatology, oncology, nutrition, exercise, and many others, now contribute to our understanding of immunity.

Environmental factors can adversely affect the immune system. These include industrial pollutants, chemicals in household products, the overuse of antibiotics and drugs, electromagnetic and other modern stresses, and the pesticides, antibiotics and other additives present in food.

As we know, the immune response can also get misdirected or out-of-proportion, as we find in the 'auto-immune' diseases. In fact, if we look at our knowledge of immunity carefully, we may begin to suspect that there is quite a bit more to know.

Because the immune response involves virtually all other systems in the body, it makes sense that if we can do things like improve digestion, excretion, and circulation, and how well we utilize oxygen, as well as how we support the body's ability to handle stress, we will improve our ability to respond to the thousand insults, every day, that are the province of the immune system.

In addition to those measures, there are nutritional substances that can facilitate and promote specific immune responses.

Here is a list of those substances:

Vitamin A is very important for the health of the mucus lining of the nose, mouth, sinuses, and stomach. People who do not get much help in fighting colds with Vitamin C, often recover quickly when given large doses of fish-liver oil Vitamin A for three to five days. Although it's possible to get too much Vitamin A in this form, it's nearly impossible to do so in the short-term. Just be sure to lower the dose once the cold has been eliminated.

Acetyl L-Carnitine, usually thought of as a brain nutrient, also facilitates metabolism in general, in its role as an oxygen carrier. It helps protect cell membranes, a key component of the immune system.

L-Arginine increases the size and activity of the thymus gland – an active element of the immune system. It benefits the liver by helping to detoxify ammonia, and prevents cirrhosis of the liver by helping liver lipid metabolism. Large doses are usually not needed to derive these benefits, and people with viral infections should avoid both supplemental arginine and foods high in this amino acid.

Astragalus has been used in traditional Chinese medicine for centuries, as a 'deep' immune booster. Echinacea, in contrast, is considered a promoter of 'superficial' immune response, working specifically on the mucous membranes. Astragalus aids adrenal function and digestion, and energizes the body by combating fatigue. It also helps protect the liver.

B-Vitamins function in many enzyme transactions, supporting the body's ability to handle stress of being ill.

Beta-1,3-glucan is the most powerful non-specific immune-activator in the nutritional field.

Bovine Colostrum helps restore the body's reservoir of immunoglobulins, a primary factor of immune system chemistry.

Bulgaricus, a friendly, transient intestinal bacteria, produces antibody-like substances, and aids the detoxification of the colon and liver.

Vitamin C reduces the frequency and intensity of winter colds, and it's now known that **Vitamin C** is involved with several hundred different important enzyme transactions in the body.

CoQ-10 helps the body to utilize oxygen. Produced in every cell of the body, it is especially important for the heart. CoQ-10 is reputed to increase the oxygen levels of the blood by as much as fifteen percent, helping to heal cancer, chronic fatigue, and other illnesses, and to prevent the recurrence of heart attacks.

DHEA (dehydroepiandrosterone) is naturally produced by the adrenal glands, and is the most abundant hormone in the human body. It improves immune function, lowers the risk of heart disease, and enhances mood, memory, and REM sleep. It aids in proper weight maintenance, and may be helpful against cancer, HIV, and lupus.

Vitamin E is an important lipid antioxidant found in every cell in the body. It helps protect the cell membranes, and prevents the oxidation of HDL cholesterol (the good kind) in the arteries.

Echinacea sales have skyrocketed in the last ten years, as more and more people have discovered how helpful it can be for fighting everything from a cold or flu, to a long-term illness like chronic fatigue. Echinacea is the single best-selling, health-promoting herb in the world.

Enzymes help in the breakdown of proteins, carbohydrates, and fats. This indirect support of the immune system is very important. Proteolytic enzymes, taken between meals, have been used as part of the treatment for many diseases, including arthritis, cancer, and other inflammatory conditions.

Essential Fatty Acids are precursors to important prostaglandins, which have a hormone-like regulatory effect on the body's response to injury and illness.

Garlic is used for high blood pressure, lice, skin troubles, worms, intestinal disorders, ulcers, and respiratory diseases. It is a nutrient-rich plant that is high in selenium, germanium, sulfur-containing amino acids, and other helpful compounds.

Garlic's antibacterial action is equivalent to one percent of penicillin. It has been used for all forms of infections (eye, ear, nose, throat, intestinal, skin, etc.). It is effective against twenty varieties of fungi, including Athlete's Foot. It has been used effectively in the treatment of candidiasis, and for thrush lesions. It also helps increase HDL cholesterol (the good kind), and lowers LDL cholesterol. It contains anti-coagulant substances that can thin the blood and help prevent heart disease and strokes, and lower blood pressure.

Germanium is a trace mineral that increases oxygen in the cells and tissues. All diseased states, or tissue degeneration, can be traced back to a common origin: hypoxia, or lack of oxygen. It induces the biosynthesis of interferons and interleukins in the immune system. It activates special cells in the thymus, which increase cancer-fighting macrophage activity. It has been used in the past with good results for people suffering from candida, viral infections, and cancer.

Goldenseal (hydrastis canadensis) is used to relieve cold and flu symptoms, aid in cases of constipation and indigestion, and to reduce skin inflammations such as eczema. Used as a mouthwash, goldenseal can help prevent gum disease, and, used as a douche, can combat vaginal infections. It is effective in digestive problems, from peptic ulcers to colitis, due to its tonic effect on the body's mucous membranes. It is a powerful anti-microbial which improves catarrhal conditions, especially those of the sinuses. It contains very powerful antibiotic-like substances, especially berberine.

Glutathione levels in the body have recently been correlated with immune strength. People with severely compromised immune systems have greatly reduced levels of glutathione. It inhibits the formation of free-radicals, and protects the cells of the immune system.

Lecithin emulsifies and promotes the transportation of fats in the body. It is the major component of all cell membranes, and is found in the protective sheath surrounding the brain, the muscles and the nerve cells. Lecithin is an inexpensive substance with major protective effects for the liver, the cardiovascular system, and the brain.

Liver has been used for strength and endurance by athletes for many years. It is also very good for keeping oneself nourished during illness, and for rebuilding after illness. Liver is a good source of B-vitamins, especially B12, and of protein.

Manganese is a necessary mineral for the functioning of the immune system. It is especially important for injuries and inflammation.

Minerals are just common sense when trying to increase immunity. They are a good way to get sufficient amounts of some of the single nutrients mentioned here, such as manganese, zinc, and Vitamins A and E.

Mushrooms, such as shiitake, maitake, and reishi fight viral infections, and build immunity. They have a long history of use in Japan and China.

NAC, or **N-Acetyl-Cysteine**, is a component of glutathione, and is a less-expensive and more effective way to raise blood levels of glutathione than taking glutathione itself. NAC helps detoxify the toxic metabolite acetylaldehyde, thereby protecting the liver.

Picrorrhiza has been used in Ayurvedic medicine for hundreds of years. It supports immune function in general, and has a specific healing and protective effect on the liver.

Probiotics such as acidophilis, bulgaricus and bifidus, are excellent nutrients to fight infections. Having good healthy intestinal bacteria is the first line of defense against harmful bacteria and viruses in food and water, and is a primary way to strengthen the immune system.

Propolis is the sticky substance that covers young buds on trees, combined with bee secretions. It has been found to have antibacterial, anti-viral, and anti-fungal activity, and enhances the body's immune response.

Pycnogenol is a patented extract from pine bark, and is a powerful free-radical scavenger -- even more powerful than well-established antioxidants such as Vitamins C and E. Because its active ingredients, proanthocyanidins, reduce inflammation by inhibiting specific protein-destroying enzymes released during the inflammatory response, they can help relieve conditions such as arthritis and sports-related injuries, and help to repair damaged collagen. Pycnogenol has been shown to protect against atherosclerosis, diabetic retinopathy, and ulcers of the digestive system.

Quercetin offers relief for hay fever and other allergic reactions. It is used to treat irritable bowel syndrome, and to help protect the intestinal lining, and aid healing.

Selenium, like Vitamin E, is an important antioxidant nutrient. In fact, when these two are taken together, their synergistic effect increases the effectiveness of each in reducing free-radicals.

Taurine, an amino acid, aids neurological function, is necessary for white blood-cell activation, and helps protect the heart and the brain.

Thymus, a small gland in the center of the chest, is an important component of the immune system. There is evidence that ingesting purified thymus in the form of certain polypeptide fractions can greatly aid the body's own production of T-cells. T-cells emerge from the thymus as highly skilled immunity factors, and help the body fight many viruses, such as hepatitis C.

Zinc is another important mineral for the immune system. It is involved with the action of many different enzymes, including the important antioxidant compound, superoxide dismutase.

HOW TO INCREASE YOUR ENERGY

Amino acids, green foods, vitamins and minerals, herbs, and other nutrients can profoundly affect energy, mood, and mental processes. Here are some nutrients that are proven ways to boost energy:

Amino Acids:

L-Carnitine is known for its ability to increase the utilization of stored body-fat, helping people to slim down and increase lean muscle mass. They also notice a significant increase in energy due to better burning of fat. L-Carnitine is also considered protective of heart function, both because the heart uses lipids as the source of most of its energy, and because it helps to reduce blood levels of fat and triglycerides. A healthy heart has a high amount of L-Carnitine present in its tissues.

L-Glutamine has many functions in the body. Recently it has been used to help heal leaky-gut syndrome and chronic immune problems, because of its importance as a fuel in the mitochondria of both the gut lining and other cells in the body. Body-builders use it because it is a primary nutrient for muscle growth. Recovering alcoholics use L-Glutamine as part of a program to help control sugar cravings and a desire for alcohol, and for mental clarity. Many healthy people find that L-Glutamine gives them similar results.

L-Phenylalanine and a related amino acid, L-Tyrosine, are precursors on the dopamine, epinephrine, and norepinephrine pathway. As such, they have been found to be helpful for depression and similar low-energy states. Although defining 'depression' apart from 'low energy' can be useful for analytical purposes, it remains true that, for all practical purposes, depression and low energy go together, and are often affected by the same body-mind disciplines.

Inosine, an amino acid metabolite, has the unique ability to increase ATP production. It is so closely related to ATP structurally that no oxygen is required for this conversion, and is the quickest pathway for the cell to get its ATP. It is closely related to the drug isoprinosine.

Vitamins:

B-Complex vitamins are important for the production of energy in many different ways. Vitamin B-1 helps both in the detoxification of toxic metabolic by-products such as acetaldehyde, and with the creation of enzymes that produce energy. When corrected, a Vitamin B-12 deficiency can yield a sudden and dramatic increase in energy. The co-enzyme form of B-12, dibencozide, sometimes works better than just the regular form. Vitamin B-6 is very important in enzyme transactions that metabolize carbohydrates, fats, and proteins. Here again, pyridoxal-5-phosphate, or P-5-P, the co-enzyme form, often gives better results. Pantothenic acid is important for helping the adrenals respond to stress, and is probably the main reason B-vitamins are considered 'stress' nutrients. Pantothene is the coenzyme that often gives better results. When experimenting with these and other B-vitamins, it is best to make sure to take a complete B-Complex in order to prevent an artificial deficiency by taking one in the absence of others.

Greens, and other Foods:

Green Algae foods Spirulina and Chlorella contain so much good, balanced nutrition, that they can hardly help from being energizing. These simple, one-celled plants are the oldest known makers of food on the planet, and they form the basis of the food chain. Using light, warmth, water and minerals, algae devote almost all their energy toward producing protein, carbohydrates, vitamins, amino acids, and other nutrients vital to life. The protein in both spirulina and chlorella is balanced, containing all the essential amino acids and most of the non-essential ones.

Spirulina grows in inland waters, so it can be farmed just like any other crop. It contains vital unsaturated fatty acids, including gamma-linolenic acid (GLA), and has many important minerals, including potassium, calcium, zinc, magnesium, selenium, iron, and phosphorus. It has vitamins, including B-12, and others of the B-Complex, E, and beta carotene, digestive enzymes, chlorophyll, and pigments that help liver function. Ounce for ounce, spirulina provides more complete protein than meat. This easily-digested protein can in itself give a boost, especially given the prevalence of high-carbohydrate diets. Since the protein in spirulina is high in phenylalanine, it has also been used as an aid to appetite suppression and weight-loss.

Chlorella has an impressive nutritional profile. Vitamins A (beta-carotene), B-l, B-2, B-3, B-6, C, E, pantothenic acid, folic acid, biotin, PABA and inositol are found in it. Minerals include calcium, magnesium, iron, zinc, iodine and phosphorus. Chlorella is the highest known source of chlorophyll, about two percent by weight -- ten times

chemicals called neurotransmitters enable the cells to talk to each other.

So far, sixty neurotransmitters have been discovered, ten of which are considered the major conductors. Here are seven common ones:

* **Acetycholine** is essential for memory and controlling movement. It is made from pantothenic acid, choline, and the energy compound ATP, produced by CoQ-10.

* **Adrenaline** and noradrenaline promote activity, alertness and mood elevation.

* **Dopamine** is essential for initiating for co-ordinating movement and sexual arousal.

* **GABA** is an inhibitory neurotransmitter for aiding concentration and chronic anxiety, and is used for patients with Parkinsonism.

* **Glycine** is also an inhibitory neurotransmitter, which with GABA, helps to prevent epilepsy.

* **Histamine** aids sensory integration in the thalamus of the brain.

* **Serotonin** is a calming counterbalance for adrenalin and noradrenalin, and induces sleep.

All of the major neurotransmitters are made from amino acids (except acetycholine). For example, glutamine is the precursor for GABA, helping with intense focal concentration and the disposal of waste ammonia, which is harmful at low levels. Tyrosine is a precursor of noradrenalin, adrenalin and dopamine, and has been used successfully in treating stress from overload or burnout. Tryptophan is a precursor of serotonin, and is converted to niacin if the body needs it.

The myelin sheath and lecithin:

Certain nerve cells are enclosed by myelin, an insulation made chiefly from fatty acids and cholesterol, which makes them capable of transmitting impulses at incredible speed. Myelin production requires linoleic acid, which is found in lecithin. Also required are the full range of amino acids, Vitamins B-2, B-3, and especially B-12, and copper and manganese.

The best brain nutrients:

Phosphatydl serine and choline, lecithin, spirulina, liver, nutritional yeast, GTF chromium, chlorella, and octaconsanol, potassium, magnesium, zinc, the B-Complex vitamins, and Vitamin C.

STRESS NUTRIENTS

Daily life is always shifting and changing. The most constant challenge is maintaining balance. The major issue always facing optimum health is the reduction of stress.

Stress is a catch-all term that takes a multitude of forms. Some are easily recognized, and others are vague and nebulous. There is physical, emotional, mental, oxidative, and environmental stress. They can come from trauma, illness, poisoning, life experiences and exercise. The one common element that all types of stress seem to share is a change in blood pH, which produces a multitude of results.

What follows is a list of nutrients that, in one or a multitude of ways, reduces stress, or aids the disarming or handling of the consequences of it. It sets out a group of categories that attempts to list, in the order of their importance, those nutrients which are most relevant to that category, though all of them are basically interchangeable.

Emotional and mental stress:

Vitamin C
B-Complex
GABA
Pregnenolone

213

L-Tryptophan or 5HTP
Bach Flower: Rescue Remedy
Melatonin
L-Tyrosine or acetyl l-tyrosine
Ginkgo
Lavender
St. John's Wort
Kava-kava
Valerian
Hops
Passion Flower
Fish oils (DHA)
Chamomile
California Poppy
Vitamin B3 (niacin)
Inositol
Vitamin B1 (thiamine)
Suma
Phosphatidyl serine
Spirulina

Physical Stress and exercise:

Vitamin C
B-Complex
L-Glutamine
L-Lysine
Royal Jelly
DMG
Magnesium
Calcium
Bee Pollen
Vitamin B5 (pantothenic acid)
Ribose
Bioflavonoids
Enzymes
Ashwaghanda
Alfalfa
Chamomile

Arnica

Oxidative and Environmental Stress:

Vitamin E
Vitamin A
Selenium
NAC (n-acetyl cysteine)
Glutathione Peroxidase
SOD (super oxide dismustase)
Methionine Reductase
Vitamin C
Alpha Lipoic acid
Astaxanthin
Bioflavonoids
B-Complex
CoQ10
Essential Fatty Acids
Acetyl l-carnitine
Enzymes
Fish Oils (EPA)
NADH
Zinc
Copper
Ginkgo
Beta 1,3 glucans
Barley Grass
Chlorella
Bilberry
Lutein
DMG

FATS AND OILS

As food becomes more processed, the meal one receives today is quite different from a hundred years ago. The results are startling.

Today, people consume much more polyunsaturated fats and oils than in the past, accounting for almost 30% of caloric intake, as opposed to an optimum level of about 4%.

Our ancestors lived on a diet with a ratio of omega-6 to omega-3 fatty acids of about 1:1. Due to massive changes in dietary habits and modern agricultural and processing procedures, the amounts of omega-3 fatty acids in foods have been dramatically reduced.

Today, this ratio is closer to 20:1 It is estimated that 85% of the population in the Western world are deficient in omega-3 fatty acids, with most getting far too much of the omega-6 fatty variety. Vegetarian diets also tend to be very high in omega-6 fatty acids.

Which fats and oils are healthful?

The polyunsaturated oils are generally from soy oil, corn oil, safflower oil and canola oil. Too much of these oils contribute to cancer and heart disease, liver and immune system problems, digestive, reproduction, weight, learning, lung, and skin problems, as well as cataracts, arthritis and premature aging.

In the past most of the fatty acids came from saturated fats and monounsaturated fats such as butter, lard, coconut oil and olive oil. Modern research now indicates that saturated fats are safer to consume than polyunsaturated fats. Saturated fats are necessary for bone health, protection of the liver, enhanced immunity, maintenance of cellular integrity, and protection of the gut from harmful microbes. They are also needed to properly utilize Essential Fatty Acids (EFA's).

The polyunsaturates in commercial vegetable oils are mostly composed of omega-6 lenoleic acid, and are low in the vital omega-3 linolenic acid. This imbalance increases the chances for creating weight gain, sterility, high blood pressure, blood clots, inflammation and cancer.

What are fats and oils?

Fats are also called lipids, which are not soluble in water. They are composed of fatty acids made up of carbon and hydrogen atoms. Most fat is in the form of triglycerides, and too much of certain fats have been linked to heart disease. Interestingly, these triglycerides are made in the liver from excess sugar, which is derived from carbohydrates, and not from fats.

There are three categories of fatty acids: **Saturated fats**, which are highly stable, unlikely to go rancid, and solid or semi-solid at room temperature. Some examples are butter, lard, coconut oil and other animal fats. **Monounsaturated fats**, which are relatively stable, unlikely to go rancid quickly, and are usually liquid at room temperature. Some examples are olive oil, peanut oil, sesame oil, and avocados. **Polyunsaturated fats** are highly reactive, go rancid easily, and remain liquid even when refrigerated. Some examples are safflower oil, corn oil, soybean oil, canola oil, flaxseed oil, cottonseed oil, and fish oils.

What are EFA's?

EFA's, or Essential Fatty Acids, are naturally-occurring unsaturated fats that are considered essential because they are not produced by the human body. There are two essential fatty acids; they are linoleic, sometimes referred to as the omega-6 fatty acid, and alpha-linolenic, referred to as the omega-3 fatty acid. Omega-3 and omega-6 fatty acids compete for the same enzymes. A proper balance of these fats in the diet is important for maintenance of good health. The best ratio appears to be 1:1.

The omega-6 and omega-3 fatty acids form different prostaglandins -- series 1,2, and 3. Prostaglandins work much like hormones do. They are involved with nearly every bodily function, including fat metabolism, inflammation, brain function, blood pressure and blood clotting. Without these essential fatty acids, several bodily functions would not be possible. The body uses linolenic acid to make two other essential fatty acids, docosahexaenoic acid (DHA), and eicosapentaenoic acid (EPA). These fatty acids are found in fish oils.

What do EFA's do?

EFA's are structural components of all cell membranes. They form hormone-like substances called prostaglandins, which are vital for almost every bodily function, including the production of steroid hormones.

Studies indicate that EFA's may increase growth hormone secretion, improve the action of insulin, enhance oxygen utilization and improve energy for optimal performance. EFA's affect total cholesterol levels and can increase levels of HDL, the good cholesterol. CLA, one of the fatty acids, appears to increase lean body mass while decreasing fat.

Low DHA levels have been linked to low serotonin levels, which are connected to an increased tendency to violence, schizophrenia, bipolar disorders, and depression. A high intake of fish protein and oils significantly decreases age-related memory loss and poor cognitive function.

Research shows EPA and DHA are crucial in the prevention of atherosclerosis, heart attack, depression, and cancer. They are also helpful for rheumatoid arthritis, ulcerative colitis, diabetes, and Raynaud's disease.

How much EFA's should be taken?

The recommended dose depends on one's genes, eating habits, and metabolism. Usually three to nine total grams per day has been shown to be sufficient. The recommend total daily intake of EPA and DHA is 650mg. to 1000mg. Fish oils utilize Vitamin E, and it is advised to add at least 100IU Vitamin E when taking them. Emulsified fish oils are best absorbed. Saturated fat intake should not exceed 8% of total calorie intake, or about eighteen grams per day. The recommended GLA daily intake is from 500mg to 1300mg per day.

What are the sources of EFA's?

The main sources of omega-6 fatty acids are vegetable oils, such as corn and soy oil, that contain a high proportion of linoleic acid. Omega-3 fatty acids are found in flaxseed oil, walnut oil, marine plankton, and fatty fish. The main component of flaxseed and walnut oils is alpha-linolenic acid, while the predominant fatty acids found in fatty fish and fish oils are eicosapentaenoic acid (EPA) and docosahexaenoic acid (DHA). Alpha-linolenic acid can be converted to EPA and DHA in the body. As we age, this ability is reduced.

What are the benefits of EFA's for pregnancy?

During pregnancy and lactation, mother's milk must supply the infants need for DHA and EPA. It is necessary for development, and the infant is unable to synthesize these essential fatty acids by itself. A deficiency of omega-3 fatty acids may result in an abnormally low birth weight, greater risk of premature birth, possible preeclampsia (pregnancy-related high blood pressure), and postpartum depression. It is recommended that women supplement 500-600mg of DHA every day during pregnancy and lactation.

Studies also indicate that low levels of omega-3 fatty acids are associated with hyperactivity in children. Early supplementation of DHA appears to reduce the risks of asthma in children.

What are the benefits of EFA's for the heart?

Studies indicate that fish oils may help prevent or reverse congestive heart failure, atherosclerosis, angina, and stroke. Fish oils reduce blood pressure, stabilize heart rhythm, and prevent blood clotting. They help maintain the elasticity of artery walls, and significantly reduce the risk of a heart attack. Fish oils are especially important for diabetics, who have an increased risk for heart disease. Daily intake of 1000mg of EPA and DHA is essential to maintaining a healthy heart.

What are some other benefits of EFA's?

Fish oils reduce inflammation and pain in rheumatoid arthritis and ulcerative colitis. Patients with ulcerative colitis generally have abnormally low blood levels of EPA. Supplementing with fish oils can reduce the severity of the condition by more than 50%.
The brain contains more than 20 grams of DHA, composing up to 20% of the cerebral cortex. DHA

composes up to 60% of the eye's retina. Fish oils help protect the brain, and nourish the skin and eyes.

GLA also has significant benefits for people who suffer from arthritis, high cholesterol, hypertension, skin conditions, weight problems, pre-menstrual syndrome (PMS), schizophrenia, and alcoholism.

What are the benefits of EFA's for cancer?

Studies indicate that high blood levels of omega-3 fatty acids, combined with low levels of omega-6 fatty acids, significantly reduces the risk of getting breast cancer. Supplementing fish oils also reduces the risks of colon and prostate cancer, while improving survival and quality of life in terminally-ill cancer patients.

What is the difference between cod liver oil and fish oils?

Cod liver oil is extracted from cod liver, and is an excellent source of Vitamins A and D. Fish oils are extracted from the flesh of fatty fish like salmon and herring, and are good sources of EPA and DHA. Fish oils contain very little Vitamin A and D, but cod liver oil does contain EPA and DHA. Cod liver oil, however, is not a good source for obtaining therapeutic amounts of

EPA and DHA, since the intake of Vitamins A and D would be too high over time.

What are some of the sources of Essential Fatty Acids (EFA's)?

Black Currant Oil is one of the most balanced oils. It contains GLA (gamma-linolenic-acid), omega-6 fatty acids, ALA (alpha-linolenic-acid), and omega-3 fatty acids. GLA helps produce PGE1 prostaglandins, hormone-like compounds that regulate cellular activity.

Borage Oil contains the highest source of GLA. It is used for reducing cholesterol, hypertension, skin conditions, weight control, pre-menstrual syndrome (PMS), and for improving joint flexibility.

Cod Liver Oil is an excellent source of Vitamins A & D. It also supplies omega-3, EPA, and DHA, but is not recommended as the primary source for DHA and EPA.

DHA (docosahexaenoic acid) is a fatty acid that is found in the gray matter of the brain and the retina of the eye. It is beneficial for mental and visual functions.

EFA (Essential Fatty Acids) are necessary for health, for rebuilding new cells, and must be obtained from the diet. They help prevent cardiovascular disease, candida, cancer, and skin disorders.

EPA (eicosapentaenoic acid) is converted from alpha-linolenic acid. EPA is converted to PGE3 prostaglandin, which helps maintain clear arteries, lower triglyceride and cholesterol levels, and to reduce high blood pressure.

Evening Primrose Oil is a very good source of GLA (d-gamma-linolenic acid). GLA supports prostaglandin function, particularly PGE1 prostaglandin, which aids skin conditions, pre-menstrual syndrome (PMS), arthritic conditions, alcoholism, mental states, and joint flexibility.

Fish Oils are a source of the omega-3 fatty acids, EPA and DHA, which help prevent atherosclerosis, heart disease, depression and cancer. They also enhance brain function and lower cholesterol levels.

Flax Oil is the best source of ALA (alpha-linolenic acid), an omega-3 fatty acid. Omega-3 fatty acids are necessary for brain function and vitality. They help protect the body from heart disease, cancer, skin problems, arthritis, and inflammation. Omega-3 produces PGE3 prostaglandin in the body. PGE3 aids in lowering cholesterol, reducing triglycerides, and maintaining healthy arteries.

GLA (d-gamma linoleic acid) is an essential fatty acid most commonly found in evening primrose oil, borage oil, black currant oil, and Mother's milk. It supports the PGE1 (prostaglandin series one) function that affects hormonal balance. GLA is used for arthritis, eczema, alcoholism, weight loss, cardiovascular disease, inflammation, brain injuries, multiple sclerosis, mental dysfunction, PMS (pre-menstrual syndrome), menopausal hot flashes, and many other conditions.

Hemp Oil is one of the most balanced oils, and is a rich source of omega-3 fatty acids. It is also high in omega-6 and omega-9 fatty acids. These essential fatty acids are important in the prevention of heart disease, arthritis, cancers, and skin problems. Hemp oil is not hallucinogenic.

Pumpkinseed Oil (curcubita pepo) is a natural source of phytosterol, beta-sitosterol, zinc, Vitamin E, selenium, and essential fatty acids. These nutrients are essential to the maintenance of a healthy prostate. Pumpkinseeds are used world-wide for the prevention and treatment of chronic prostatic hypertrophy.

Salmon Oil is a rich source of omega-3 fatty acids, especially EPA and DHA, which are known to lower cholesterol, lower blood pressure, prevent heart disease and arthritis. They also protect the brain and nourish the skin and eyes.

ENZYMES AND THE DIGESTIVE SYSTEM

Enzymes occur naturally in all living things. All life processes consist of a complex series of chemical reactions called metabolism. Enzymes are the catalysts that make metabolism possible. They play important roles in breathing, digestion, growth, blood coagulation, and reproduction. We get enzymes in food, but much of our food is enzyme-deficient because it has been cooked, processed, or sprayed with preservatives, pesticides, insecticides and other enzyme killers.

Enzymes are necessary for digestion and for the burning of food in the body. Digestion begins in the mouth with the secretion of amylase, and in the stomach with the release of pepsin, hydrochloric acid and bile. Enzymes are particularly important in the duodenum, the first part of the small intestine.

Food generally consists of three basic groups: proteins, fats, and carbohydrates. To digest protein we need proteolytic enzymes, for fats we need lipolytic enzymes, and for carbohydrates, amylolytic enzymes. There are many other enzymes for specific food nutrients. For example, intestinal bloating, gas, or diarrhea from milk products may be due to a lack of the enzyme, lactase, which breaks down lactose, or milk sugar, so it will not ferment in the colon.

Enzyme supplements are made from plant and animal sources. Pancreatin (containing protease, amylase, and lipase), chymotrypsin, and trypsin are made from hog or ox pancreas. Other enzyme supplements are extracted from plants, including bromelain (from pineapple), papain (from papaya), and ficin (from fig). Bromelain and papain are an aid in the digestion of protein. Amylolytic enzymes are from cereal grains. Some enzymes are bacterial or fungal in origin ('microbial'), and are derived from fermentation processes involving fungi, or from bacteria such as aspergillus oryzae and aspergillus niger.

Enzymes aid in the relief of gas, indigestion, intestinal and systemic toxicity, skin blemishes, and digestive disorders. Enzymes used for acute and chronic conditions are called 'systemic enzyme therapy'. These enzymes are protected from the stomach's acid, and are designed to work in the small intestine. Systemic enzyme therapy has shown great promise in fighting inflammation, arthritis, cancer, circulatory disorders, sports injuries, multiple sclerosis, HIV/AIDS, and other conditions. Often, these are proteolytic enzymes that are taken unaccompanied by food.

The body's enzyme supply decreases in quantity and activity with aging. Enzyme production is also reduced by poor diet, illness, injury, environmental toxins, and stress. Enzymes help slow the aging process. Co-enzymes (or co-factors) such as vitamins, trace minerals, and minerals are essential for the activity of many enzymes. For example, there are over three hundred enzymes in the human body that require the trace mineral, zinc, to function properly. Some enzymes may require B vitamins, magnesium, iron, copper, and selenium. Adding enzymes to a good supplement program, or adding supplements to an enzyme program, insures positive results.

HERBAL GLOSSARY

Alterative: Changes present nutritive and excretory processes to regulate body functions.

Analgesic: Used orally to relieve pain.

Anodyne: Used externally to relieve pain.

Antibiotic: Stops the growth of microorganisms.

Antihydropic: Flushes out excess body fluid.

Anti-inflammatory: Reduces inflammation.

Antiperiodic: Counteracts periodic diseases.

Antipyretic: Reduces fevers.

Antiseptic: Eliminates harmful bacteria.

Antispasmodic: Relieves cramps, spasms and coughs.

Antisyphilic: Fights venereal disease.

Aperient: Stimulates and purges the bowels.

Aphrodisiac: Strengthens sexual desire and potency.

Appetizer: Increases the appetite.

Aromatic: Activates the gastrointestinal system, and has a strong smell or taste.

Astrigent: Contracts, and reduces or stops, discharges.

Calmative: Calms the nerves.

Cardiac: Strengthens the heart and cardiovascular system.

Carminative: Expels digestive gas.

Cathartic: Works as a laxative.

Cholagogue: Increases the flow of bile.

Demulcent: Soothes inflammation of internal organs.

Depurant: Stimulates elimination and purifies the blood.

Diaphoretic: Activates perspiration.

Digestant: Aids digestion.

Diuretic: Increases the flow of urine.

Emmenagogue: Increases menstrual flow.

Emetic: Induces vomiting.

Emollient: Softens and strengthens the skin.

Expectorant: Expels mucus from the lungs and bronchial system.

Febrifuge: Reduces fevers.

Germicide: Destroys pathogenic microorganisms.

Hemostatic: Stops bleeding.

Hepatic: Tones the liver and increases the flow of bile.

Hormonal: Contains natural hormones.

Laxative: Stimulates bowel movements.

Nervine: Strengthens and heals the nerves.

Purgative: Purges and cleans the bowels.

Relaxant: Calms the nervous system.

Sedative: Reduces anxiety, nervousness and distress.

Stimulant: Stimulates internal organs.

Stomachic: Strengthens the stomach and increases appetite.

Styptic: Stops bleeding by contracting blood vessels.
Sudorific: Stimulates perspiration.
Tonic: Increases energy and tone.
Vermicide: Kills worms and parasites.
Vermifuge: Expels worms and parasites.
Vulnerary: Promotes healing.
Vasoconstrictor: Shrinks blood vessels and capillaries.

THE REGULATION
CONTROVERSY

Frequently, the Food and Drug
Administration (FDA) and the news
media have projected a picture of a
dietary supplement marketplace that
is unregulated and dangerous for the
consumer -- this is inaccurate. The
major problem between the health
supplement industry and the FDA
pivots on the FDA being drug-
oriented, pharmaceutically staffed,
and committed to the protection of
the drug industry if a nutrient poses a
threat to the sale of a drug in the
marketplace.

In 1989, the FDA banned L-
tryptophan from the marketplace
after one contaminated batch
containing e-coli bacteria caused
serious illness and deaths. The
dietary supplement industry
responded immediately and issued
recalls. The Japanese manufacturer
never made tryptophan again, and no
further problems occurred. The FDA
could have temporarily stopped sales
of L-tryptophan until the problem
had been resolved (as it did with
Tylenol when deaths occurred due to
contamination). Instead, L-
tryptophan was banned from the
marketplace. At the time, L-
tryptophan had become the number
one product in the marketplace for
economical effective, safe, non-
habit-forming sleeping pills. The

ban was lifted in 1996, when L-tryptophan was made available to the public at a dramatically higher price (from 23 cents per gram to an exorbitant 25 dollars per gram) and by prescription only.

More recently, the FDA attempted to control the marketplace by stating that it had authority over substances that dealt with disease, and went on to list such conditions as pregnancy, menopause, and weight control as diseases. The courts of this country however have reprimanded the FDA for its actions to restrict natural products from the marketplace.

The fact that nutrients do have an effect on disease is overwhelmingly documented. Information that certain dietary supplements have an effect on a disease must come from third-party literature, and not directly from the company marketing the product. The FDA has the power to sue any company that makes a claim that a product cures or treats a disease.

The Dietary Supplement Health and Education Act (DSHEA) was unanimously passed by Congress in 1994. This law created a new category different from foods or drugs. The category is dietary supplements: vitamins, minerals, amino acids, herbs, and botanicals. Congress intended this law to create a reasonable regulatory framework to benefit the over 110 million Americans who consume dietary supplements. The goal was to protect access to, and information about, dietary supplements.

The DSHEA legislation increased the FDA's regulatory powers. The FDA has always been able to seize any dietary supplement that poses a health risk, but now the FDA can require dietary supplements to meet strict manufacturing requirements, including potency, cleanliness, and stability. The FDA can obtain an injunction against the sale of any dietary supplement that presents false or unsubstantiated claims, and can charge any company selling a dietary supplement that is toxic or unsanitary with a criminal offense.

Most dietary supplement manufacturers in today's marketplace are pharmaceutically licensed, responsible, and meet strict manufacturing requirements. The products on the shelves of vitamin and health food stores today represent a tremendous effort on the part of an industry committed to creating and maintaining the health of the purchaser.

The dietary supplement industry demonstrates a virtually religious fervor in its desire to aid people's health. This industry provides dramatic economic benefits to society at large, which result from the use of its products. It has met the challenges of the last fifteen years, and has succeeded in developing the highest standards. It has organized an appraisal of itself as an industry, and can be proud of its heritage and accomplishments against overwhelming odds and vehement criticism.

In the passing years, the major suppliers of dietary supplements have developed excellent, responsible formulations. They have provided training regarding their products, and have developed a market that reaps the benefits from an industry committed to scientific research and information. The dietary supplement industry brings freedom of choice into the marketplace. It provides the individual with power over his or her own well-being by offering the public access to nutritional information and products that improve and maintain optimal health.

About the Author:

Michael LeVesque, is a teacher, health advocate, and entrepreneur. For the past 31 years, he has written numerous articles and commentaries on health issues. He extensively uses nutritional supplements, reads nutritional science, and is an advocate of alternative natural medicines. His areas of specialization include nutrition for brain function, the immune system, and disease prevention. He hosts a Website on nutritional issues at:

www.VitaminsInAmerica.com.

Michael is President and CEO of the five largest independent vitamin stores in the San Francisco Bay Area. He is one of the first health supplement retailers with a presence on the internet.